The Future of Healthcare: Global Trends Worth Watching

ACHE Management Series Editorial Board

Your board, staff, or clients may also benefit from this book's insight. For more information on quantity discounts, contact the Health Administration Press Marketing Manager at (312) 424–9470.

This publication is intended to provide accurate and authoritative information in regard to the subject matter covered. It is sold, or otherwise provided, with the understanding that the publisher is not engaged in rendering professional services. If professional advice or other expert assistance is required, the services of a competent professional should be sought.

The statements and opinions contained in this book are strictly those of the authors and do not represent the official positions of the American College of Healthcare Executives or the Foundation of the American College of Healthcare Executives.

Library of Congress Cataloging-in-Publication Data

Garman, Andrew N.
  The future of healthcare : global trends worth watching / Andrew N. Garman,
Tricia J. Johnson, and Thomas C. Royer.
       p. cm.
  Includes bibliographical references.
  ISBN 978-1-56793-379-6 (alk. paper)
  1. Medical care—Forecasting. 2. Medical innovations. 3. Globalization.
I. Johnson, Tricia J. II. Royer, Thomas C. III. Title.
  RA425.G195 2011
  362.101'12—dc22

                              2010052575

The paper used in this publication meets the minimum requirements of American National Standard for Information Sciences—Permanence of Paper for Printed Library Materials, ANSI Z39.48-1984. ⊗™

Acquisitions editor: Eileen Lynch; Project manager: Jennifer Seibert; Cover illustration: Sean Kane; Cover designer: Scott Miller; Layout: BookComp; Printer: Cushing-Malloy

Found an error or a typo? We want to know! Please e-mail it to hap1@ache.org, and put "Book Error" in the subject line.

For photocopying and copyright information, please contact Copyright Clearance Center at www.copyright.com or at (978) 750–8400.

Health Administration Press
A division of the Foundation of the American
   College of Healthcare Executives
One North Franklin Street, Suite 1700
Chicago, IL 60606–3529
(312) 424–2800

CHAPTER 1

Introduction

CHANGE IN THE UNITED STATES

The United States recently signed into law its most sweeping health reform bill since Medicare was enacted in 1965. Most of the press attention has been on the effects these changes will have on healthcare in the United States. For the foreseeable future, these changes will be the day-to-day focus of most healthcare managers. Most consumers in the United States, however, will not care where the legislation came from or how it changes payments to providers and regulation of insurance companies. Mainly they will want to know the effect it will have on their ability to access the providers they need when they need them and their out-of-pocket costs.

So what does the future hold? While there are many questions that only time will answer, in the public opinion a few things do seem certain: Without a sense of the broader context of these reforms, consumers may feel that the decisions were recklessly made; without an understanding of other care models, consumers will readily fear horror stories about such issues as "death panels" and six-month waiting lists; and without clarity on the difference between costs and value, they will perceive any effort to hold down costs no differently than efforts to ration care.

Realistically, most of the proposed changes stem from programs and processes with a demonstrated track record somewhere else. For the first time, "somewhere else" is outside US borders. These programs and processes have not been discussed much in the media, and for good reason: They often involve a depth of complexity through which few consumers care to wade. Most consumers do not want to learn about economics, geography, and world cultures just to understand where healthcare is going. They simply want good care so they can go on living their lives. Healthcare managers, however, need to understand

where these changes are coming from—now and in the future.

FINDING THE ISLANDS OF TRUTH (IN A SEA OF MISINFORMATION)

Throughout this book, we strive to find the most reliable information we can to support our points. The most reliable sources have a vested interest in the accuracy of the data rather than their implications. Agenda-free data are difficult to find, cumbersome to organize, and tricky to interpret. As such they do not often find their way into press releases and news articles, but they are worth the trouble to track down for the clarity they can provide.

For example, consider *medical travel*—travel to other countries for purposes of obtaining medical care (Garman, Milstein, and Anderson 2008). The casual US reader may have first picked up this story in 2007/2008, when articles citing the statistic that approximately 150,000 Americans traveled overseas for healthcare in 2006 started appearing in magazines such as *Forbes* (Cooperman 2007). Most articles did not provide a source for this number, while others attributed the figure to secondary sources, such as the American Medical Association (e.g., Newsome 2008). So where did this statistic come from? It was a guess by Josef Woodman, author of *Patients Beyond Borders*, a book promoting medical tourism, based on his conversations with hospital administrators from other countries. He reckoned half traveled over the southern borders for dental and plastic surgery and half traveled overseas for major procedures (Woodman 2007; Freyer 2007).

Not long after Woodman's book was published, the story grew, and the sources became more mainstream. By winter, NBC had quoted the number as 500,000 and the travel as *overseas*. This new estimate was attributed to research by the National Coalition on Health Care (NCHC), a well-respected not-for-profit organization focused on health system reform, a seemingly more reliable source. The problem was that NCHC never conducted a study on medical travel.

Several consulting firms soon stepped in with estimates that were more rigorous but also wildly different. The McKinsey authors pegged their inpatient-only estimate at 60,000 to 85,000 patients per year (Ehrbeck, Guevara, and Mango 2008); Deloitte's more comprehen-sive estimate was 750,000 (Keckley and Underwood 2008). These analyses were proprietary, so no follow-up efforts were made to reconcile the differences, and as you might guess, the Deloitte number tended to be the one that was circulated in the headlines. As of this writing, the estimates are still rising. A 2009 article in *Healthcare Financial Management*, citing "data from several sources" as its basis, concluded that "as many as 2 million Americans went abroad for healthcare" in 2008 (Bauer 2009, 36). (To the author's defense, he did include a caveat that the sources he included in the article provided "rough estimates at best." Our prediction is that his number will be quoted but not his caveat.)

DISCOVERING THE IMPLICATIONS FOR YOUR ORGANIZATION

In this book we draw many conclusions about where we are likely headed in the coming years. In some cases our conclusions may one day seem prophetic; in other cases forces will intervene to change the direction of these trends. Our hope is that this book points you in useful directions and provokes you to think about the ways your organization can prepare for changing demands and opportunities. To this end, Chapter 2 focuses on how innovations emerge and spread. If you understand these phenomena, you will be in the best position to interpret the meaning of trends. The following chapters identify the trends shaping healthcare today and their implications. The book concludes with two appendixes of additional resources. Appendix 1 lists authoritative sources available on the Web for tracking global trends across a variety of key indicators.

Appendix 2 describes the "futures task force" approach that CHRISTUS Health, one of the largest Catholic healthcare systems in the United States, has taken in response to macro-level trends and their implications for its charitable mission. As the approach illustrates, discussions about the future are often as much about education and awareness-building as they are about the organization's plans; both ingredients are essential to organizational resilience and growth.

CHAPTER 2

How Innovations Emerge and Spread

Tracking trends in healthcare across the globe could easily become a full-time job. Models of innovation are tools you can use to sort out the most important trends. Two models—the Disruptive Innovation model and the Diffusion of Innovation model—are particularly useful in considering the future of specific innovations. Both have been used extensively, though they are often misunderstood and misapplied. This chapter will describe these models and their applications.

THE DISRUPTIVE INNOVATION MODEL

Pioneered by Clayton Christensen, the Disruptive Innovation (DI) model can be used to evaluate the threat of new entrants into an existing product or service space (Christensen, Bohmer, and Kenagy 2000). The model is most easily explained through the use of graphs illustrating changes in performance expectations over time. The first graph in Exhibit 2.1 includes two lines: The top line tracks the expectations of the most demanding customers of a particular product or service over time, and the bottom line tracks the same trend for the least demanding customers. In the case of healthcare services, the top line might represent the highly engaged patient, one who is well informed about his health and brings specific questions to the medical visit and expectations about what he will take away from it. Patients represented by the lower line, in contrast, have fewer expectations about the service encounter and may require less of providers in the way of customized care or special services. Patients who are relatively healthy and highly functional might fit this description, as would patients who are particularly good at self-managing their conditions.

In healthcare and every other sector, dominant providers tend to emerge over time. This trend is depicted in the second graph. You'll notice the slope of this new line is steeper than the customer lines. The reason is that, in a competitive environment, organizations focus on keeping ahead of their competitors. Inevitably, this competition also leads these organizations to innovate in anticipation of what customers might ask for in the future. (I [AG] have referred to this competitive effect as the "peanut butter and jelly in the same jar" phenomenon.) This race to invent and deploy value-added services and products eventually outpaces what customers want—and want to pay for.

As the costs of the dominant providers' innovations continue to escalate, the least demanding customers become increasingly interested in finding lower-cost options to meet their needs. This demand opens an opportunity for new organizations to enter the market, which is represented by the line depicted in the third graph (page 8). Typically these new entrants find their footing by providing products/services that the lower-demand customers view as good enough and at a much lower cost.

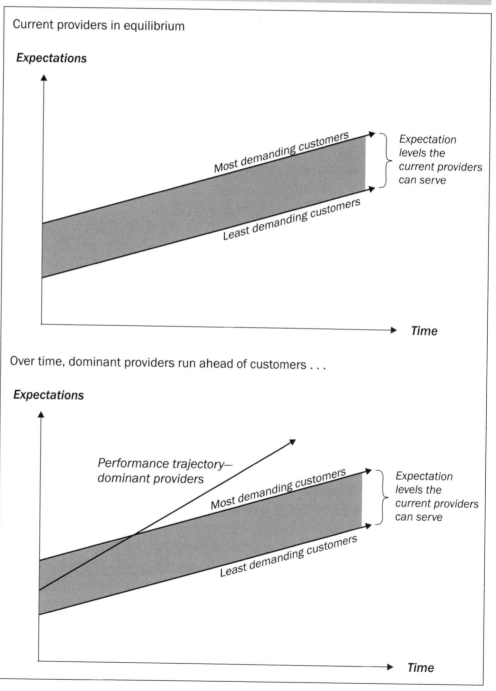

EXHIBIT 2.1: Performance Expectations Over Time

Current providers in equilibrium

Expectations

Most demanding customers

Least demanding customers

Expectation levels the current providers can serve

Time

Over time, dominant providers run ahead of customers . . .

Expectations

Performance trajectory—dominant providers

Most demanding customers

Least demanding customers

Expectation levels the current providers can serve

Time

(continued)

... opening up opportunities for higher-efficiency providers.

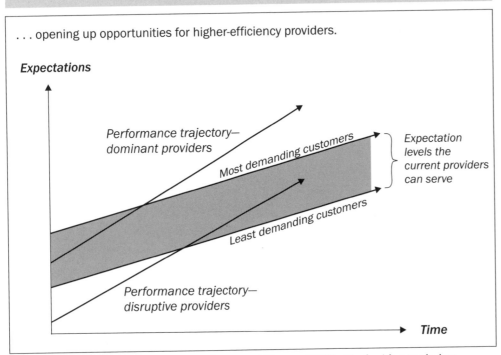

SOURCE: Adapted from Christensen, Bohmer, and Kenagy (2000). Used with permission.

Although the model originated in manufacturing, it has since proven to be relevant to many other industries, including healthcare. Familiar examples of disruptive providers in recent years include ambulatory surgical centers and retail clinics. The model is particularly useful in considering the prospect of new entrants because it includes a specific set of criteria by which the threat of new entrants can be assessed. The questions in the following checklist are based on those criteria:

1. Is the business model of the new entrant simpler and/or less costly? Is the initial focus an underserved market?

2. Are the products/services of the new entrant sufficient in the eyes of consumers? They may contain fewer or even lower-quality features, as long as the consumers find them acceptable.

3. Are there organizational or regulatory barriers that once protected the dominant providers but are

being successfully challenged by the new entrant?

4. Will mainstream consumers eventually be able to access these products/services without fundamentally changing their buying patterns?

If your answer to all four of these questions is "yes," there is potential for a market disruption. If your answer to one or more is "no," the likelihood that a new organization will enter the market is much less—today, anyway. Therefore, we add a fifth question to the checklist:

5. What is the most likely pathway to turning any/all of the above "no" answers into "yes" answers? Who is most likely to pursue this opportunity, what kinds of resources would they need, and how long would it take?

Example Application: Medical Travel

As we noted in Chapter 1, press coverage of US patients traveling overseas for care has been considerable, particularly in the years leading up to healthcare reform. Although people had traveled to other countries for years for cosmetic procedures, "medical tourism" seemed to be morphing into a broader trend

of traveling to other countries for medically essential services from lower-cost providers. Without hard data to guide them, journalists bid up each other's estimates to the point where we were reading unsubstantiated claims that 2 million patients per year were traveling out of the United States for medical care. Although our own analyses suggest that the volumes were considerably lower (Johnson and Garman 2010), the trend was clearly robust, so we wondered whether medical tourism providers (MTPs) might be forming into a disruptive innovation to the US healthcare system.

To consider this possibility, let's apply the checklist questions in order. Question #1: The business model of international providers is often more straightforward than that of US nonprofit hospitals, which are tightly regulated by a breadth of agencies and have responsibilities to their local communities and charitable missions. MTPs marketed to uninsured patients, so they were targeting an underserved market. Thus, the answer to question #1 was "yes."

Question #2, which concerns consumers' perception of the services, poses our first hurdle to disruption. How many potential consumers view hospitals in other countries as sufficient for their needs? Here the early media stories about medical tourists are particularly telling. The prototypical medical travelers interviewed for these stories were relatively sophisticated consumers. They had thoughtful and well-reasoned answers to why they chose to travel for care; they also tended to earn higher incomes and were already travel savvy. It would be challenging for MTPs to reach consumers beyond these more sophisticated early adopters. To address these concerns, MTPs took various steps, including obtaining internationally recognizable accreditations (e.g., Joint Commission International) and developing sophisticated "door-to-door" concierge operations to eliminate perceived uncertainties related to international travel. So, the answer to question #2 was "maybe."

Question #3 considers regulatory barriers. In this area MTPs had some key competitive advantages. Many operated in countries that did not have the same levels of regulatory oversight that their US counterparts had. Quality implications aside, the ability to operate outside of these regulatory structures fit the definition of "challenging existing entry barriers." Thus, we had another "yes."

The answer to question #4, which concerns the mainstream consumer, was a clear "no." Attracting patients with no other choices was one matter; attracting patients who had a viable local option was another. Few patients with the means to choose would opt to travel out of the country for care, unless there were strong incentives to do so—and even then, most would still choose to stay home (Milstein and Smith 2007).

Tallying these responses, we answered "yes" twice, "maybe" once, and "no" once (see Exhibit 2.2), so medical tourism did not appear to be an emerging disruptive innovation—at least not at that point in time. Now let's consider the pathway in question #5. For this one, let's imagine that an MTP *could* be viewed as fully comparable to a US provider, eliminate the barriers that currently prevent traveling for care, shrink the distance people need to travel, and fully integrate its services into a mainstream health plan. What would that arrangement look like? Thinking this question through a bit, we hit upon the prospect of the *domestic* MTP as a potentially disruptive force. We pick this topic up again in Chapter 4.

ROGERS'S DIFFUSION OF INNOVATION MODEL

Although the Christensen DI model can be a terrific tool for assessing

EXHIBIT 2.2: Assessment of Medical Travel as a Potentially Disruptive Innovation

Criterion	Yes	Maybe	No
Simpler/less costly business model	☑	☐	☐
Product/service sufficient in the eyes of the consumer	☐	☑	☐
New entrant successfully challenges organizational/regulatory barriers	☑	☐	☐
Mainstream consumers can eventually access product/service without changing buying patterns	☐	☐	☑

market competitors, other models are useful for evaluating the prospects for innovations that do not necessarily disrupt the markets within which they spread. The most widely recognized among them is the Diffusion of Innovation model, pioneered by Everett Rogers (1995). The model is best known for its description of the spread of innovations as four distinct phases: innovators (roughly the first 2.5 percent), early adopters (the next 13.5 percent), early majority (the next 34 percent), late majority (the following 34 percent), and the laggards (the final 16 percent). While much has been made in the popular press of the characteristics of people

and organizations who tend to adopt during each phase, in many ways the real value of the model is its usefulness in assessing the potential for a given innovation to move from the pilot stage to something the rest of healthcare world needs to reckon with. To explain how these diffusions operate, we must first discuss the appropriate level of analysis. Exhibit 2.3 provides examples of some of these key levels and how Rogers's phases add up in real numbers.

Keeping in mind that the cutoffs where one phase ends and another begins are far less important than the overall shape these trends tend to take, let's look at an example.

EXHIBIT 2.3: Diffusion at Different Levels of Analysis

	Level of Analysis			
Stage of Diffusion	US Hospitals[1] (5,815)	US Academic Medical Centers[2] (122)	US States (50)	Countries in the OECD Health Database[3] (34)
Innovators	0–145	0–3	0–1	0–1
Early adopters	146–930	4–19	2–8	2–5
Early majority	931–2,908	20–61	9–25	6–17
Late majority	2,909–4,885	62–103	26–42	18–28
Laggards	4,889+	104+	43+	29+

SOURCES: Data from [1]American Hospital Association (2009); [2]University HealthSystem Consortium (2010); [3]OECD (2010d).

Case Example: Country-Level Adoption of Patient Classification Systems

Throughout this book we describe innovations happening in other countries that may find their way to the United States. Which are most likely to affect our healthcare system, and how long might they take? We can look at one of our more important health system exports—patient classification systems—for some clues. The data for this example come from the last chapter of *The Globalization of Managerial Innova-tion in Health Care* (D'Aunno, Kimberly, and de Pouvourville 2008) and represent the first year in which a US-style classification system was investigated for adoption by other countries. Using the countries in the Organisation for Economic Co-operation and Development (OECD) database as our level of analysis, we'd expect to see upticks after the first two or so countries and again after the first six or so (see Exhibit 2.4). The time between adoption of the system by the first country (the United States) and adoption by the third is roughly 14 years (as levels of analysis expand, so do the time horizons associated with diffusion). The time between adoption by the third country and adoption by the seventh is four years. The Early Adopter phase ended in the late 1980s, and we are now in the Early Majority phase. As the graph shows, the pace of uptick has begun to slow in more recent years.

In addition to identifying phases of innovation, Rogers's work also addresses key factors related to the pace of its diffusion, including the communications necessary to support it, the social system in which it takes place, and the effects of time. For our purposes, characteristics of the innovation are particularly salient. Rogers's checklist includes the following questions:

EXHIBIT 2.4: Total Countries Investigating or Adopting Patient Classification Systems by Year

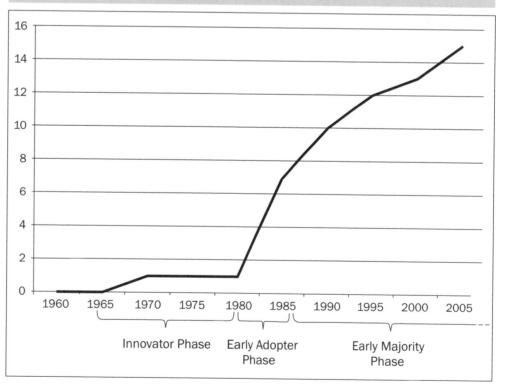

1. Can the innovation provide *relative advantage*? In other words, could adopting the innovation make a clear and visible difference to consumers?

2. Is the innovation *compatible* with the organization considering its adoption? In other words, does it appear to be congruent with the current values and needs of the people responsible for its adoption?

3. Is the innovation relatively *simple*? Is adoption possible without major changes?

4. Is the innovation "*trialable*"? Can it be pilot tested and adapted to local needs before a more substantial commitment is made?

5. Are the innovation and its benefits *readily observable*? Can they be viewed or experienced by the people who would adopt them?

Diffusion is more likely to occur to the extent that an innovation has these properties. However, having all of these properties does not guarantee that the innovation will spread—particularly in healthcare. To explain why, we need to consider the context in which we operate.

Much adaptation in healthcare is a response to rule changes. For example, we may learn that reimbursements are going to change over time; in response, we model the effects these changes will have on our organizations as best we can, weigh our options for adapting to these new realities, and select the adaptive measures we think will work best. Within this sort of context, innovations tend to flow only toward the pressures we are facing.

At the level of a national healthcare system, the same rules of innovation diffusion can be applied. As one system begins to look more like other systems, the barriers to diffusion begin to break down. Although the US healthcare system remains unique in the world in many ways, health reform will add some elements that are similar to those of other countries' health systems. As a result, the opportunities to benefit from innovations from other countries will also increase. We pick up this topic again when we discuss convergence and harmonization in Chapter 7.

CHAPTER 3

The Changing Nature of Health Information

I n the winter of 2008, I (AG) had the opportunity to interview "Jane," an uninsured patient who was recovering from surgery in a Joint Commission International–accredited hospital in southeast Asia. Originally from the United States, she had been driving trucks for a private-sector contractor in Iraq prior to her surgery; the job paid well and it didn't take long for her to save up enough money to afford the procedure. When I asked her how she came to hear of this hospital, she told me about numerous Internet groups that focus on finding providers for certain kinds of surgeries. The hospital she selected had been highly recommended by someone she had met and corresponded with through one of the sites.

This patient's demographic—female American truck drivers working in Iraq in 2008—probably has a greater-than-average risk tolerance. Nevertheless, the example illustrates some fundamental realities that are important to keep in mind as the field continues its health information evolution. Chief among these developments is the role of social comparison in decision making. When choosing providers, people are likely to continue to go with personal referrals rather than hard facts. We will return to this theme later in the chapter; for now, consider the following key trends.

TRANSPARENCY OF CARE QUALITY

There is a clear trend toward greater availability of "outcomes" data, as well as toward payers' use of these data to reward providers for quality of care. The outcomes of interest differ among stakeholders. For the consumer, they might be quality of life, restoration of health, or simply feeling better. For a physician, they might be whether there were post-procedure complications, whether the patient left the hospital alive, or whether the patient survived 30 days post-hospitalization. These varying definitions of "outcomes" make it difficult to report them in ways that will be most meaningful to the different consumers involved. We are still early in this process, and approaches are likely to continue to evolve in the coming years. Regardless, the trend toward using these data to guide decision making is here to stay and seems poised to continue growing.

GREATER USE OF THE INTERNET IN HEALTH DECISION MAKING

In 2009, approximately 61 percent of American adults reported that they look online for health information—up from 25 percent just a decade earlier (Fox and Jones 2009). The majority of these consumers turn primarily to health professionals, friends, and family members for health advice; however, more than 40 percent of these online health consumers reported reading user-generated health information—commentaries posted online in reviews, blogs, forums, and message boards.

Consumers turning to the Internet for health information face an overwhelming number of available sites. As we write this book, a simple search for "heart failure" yields 16.9

million results in Google; narrowing the search to "heart failure treatment" still returns 12.4 million hits. Sifting through online information is challenging, to say the least, and the sites that receive the most traffic will be those with the most marketing savvy, not necessarily the most reliable data. For example, a study by the market research firm comScore found that in the three months after the H1N1 outbreak, more than four times as many Web searchers clicked through to Wikipedia than to the Centers for Disease Control and Prevention—and one of the top five sites in this search wasn't even a medical or news site; it was Clorox's (Abraham 2010). Even the savviest consumers can easily get lost looking for reliable, objective information on healthcare quality. To address the need for quality information about providers, advocacy sites such as Consumer Reports and business sites such as Angie's List have developed substantial online programs. We anticipate that this trend will continue—and accelerate—to the point where all major online search and advertising companies offer competitive services. This movement will also support another major trend: personal health information.

THE POWER OF PERSONAL HEALTH INFORMATION

As we write this book, the electronic health record story that many US healthcare providers are preoccupied with is "meaningful use." While these providers are taking advantage of a time-limited opportunity to find outside support for electronic health record implementation, the early adopters are experimenting with the next level of value that can be derived from this opportunity: greater use of electronic health data for large-scale applications, such as genetic studies and efficiency analyses. However, the role of the consumer—particularly with regard to greater data access—may take us to even more interesting places.

In the winter of 2008, Google announced a pilot program in collaboration with Cleveland Clinic that would give consumers greater access to and control over health information. Soon afterward, Microsoft announced partnerships that would enable consumers to import information into its personal health record application, HealthVault, from health insurers and academic medical centers. In each case, press releases announced that the projects improved consumer access as well as the portability of health information. What was not discussed, and is not yet receiving the attention it deserves, is the fundamental change this access introduces in terms of consumers' relationships with their care providers. There has been plenty of discussion about the privacy implications stemming from the Health Insurance Portability and Accountability Act (i.e., How can patient data be safeguarded once the patients leave the hospital?) and about the integrity of the data (e.g., Will patients be able to modify their records and, if so, in what ways and to what ends?), but little about the change's effect on the patient–provider relationship.

To understand the magnitude of this change, consider all of the reasons you see a doctor, a nurse, or another care provider. For many people, a visit is driven either by prevention (the annual checkup) or by a concern (a set of symptoms or questions). What services does the clinician provide? In both cases, she typically performs some diagnostics—a weight and blood pressure check, for example—and there is some exchange of opinions or recommendations. Now imag-

ine you are going to the doctor not with a list of questions but with your own six-month record of your weight, blood pressure, and other measures. Now let's take one step further: What if software could provide you with the same analysis the clinician could, but at a more convenient time and at a lower cost? This capability would cause a fundamental shift toward increased patient ownership and responsibility for treatment choices.

We believe that many people (not all, but many) would balk at the idea of giving up an opportunity for a human interaction to discuss their health in favor of using a computerized expert system. Herein lies the key point: It's highly possible that the future will see technical expertise becoming more the commodity and service the key differentiator.

ELECTRONIC HEALTH RECORDS: LINKING PROVIDERS

The Patient Protection and Affordable Care Act provides substantial financial incentives to healthcare providers to adopt electronic medical records. The United States is far behind some countries with regard to the connectivity of patient health information. The short-term goal is to link providers—primary care physicians, specialists, hospitals, imaging centers, and other practitioners anywhere in the country—through a seamless sharing of health information.

This same connectivity could readily extend beyond US borders. Physicians in the United States will soon be able to seamlessly and virtually consult, for example, with a primary care physician in the United Arab Emirates about patients who traveled to the United States for care, thus providing more seamless care to our international patients. US consumers who travel abroad for care will also receive better care because of the ability of the physician in the destination hospital to virtually consult with the patient's primary care provider in the United States.

IMPLICATIONS

Let's apply these trends to a patient in a hypothetical future state. In this future we see Mary, who has a chronic condition and wants to find a good doctor to manage her treatment. Mary searches the Web and finds several social networking sites for people with similar conditions. Instead of anonymous postings, she finds links to personal pages. She posts her question to the group, with the subject "Seeking referral for a doctor in Chicago," and several local people respond to her directly with their recommendations. They all have nice things to say, but the message that really sways her is Jill's. Not only does Jill explain in detail about how her doctor helped her; she also takes a step that today might seem unthinkable: She gives Mary the link to her online medical record, where she can review the care plan for herself.

CHAPTER 4

Traveling for Value

IS US HEALTHCARE IN A TRADE DEFICIT?

From an economic perspective, identification of the factors driving inbound and outbound travel for medical care is critically important at both the national level, with President Obama's National Export Initiative to double exports by 2015, and at the individual provider level, where relatively small changes in the number of patients can have substantial revenue implications.

How many people do in fact travel for care? Although there are no official statistics, objective attempts at measurement have estimated that in 2007 between 50,300 and 121,400 people from other countries traveled into the United States, and between 42,600 and 102,900 Americans traveled outside the United

States, for medical care that required an inpatient hospital stay (Johnson and Garman 2010). These and other estimates suggest that the United States remains a net exporter of health services. People traveling into the United States spent between $489 million (M) and $1.2 billion (B) on care, while those leaving the United States spent $87M to $209M on care in other countries.

As with many other goods and services, however, the dollars tell only half of the story. Had these value-conscious US patients not left the country and instead received care domestically, they could have represented an additional $579M to $1.4B in local patient care.

WHAT DOES TRAVELING FOR VALUE MEAN?

Value is a measure of the relationship between the cost and quality of healthcare: the higher the quality relative to the cost, the higher the value. Higher-value healthcare can refer to care that is (1) lower cost, for the same quality level; (2) higher quality for the same cost; or (3) both higher quality and lower cost. The concept of value-driven healthcare is not new, but the idea of *traveling* for value-driven healthcare has

gained attention only recently, first with international medical travel and now with medical travel within the United States. Traveling for value is predicated on the consumer's ability to compare both quality and costs; comparisons of only one of these two factors provide an incomplete picture of value.

There is no debate that healthcare costs in the United States are the highest in the developed world, both as a proportion of the gross domestic product (GDP) and per capita, and that these costs have outpaced the growth of GDP. In response to high and increasing healthcare costs, individual out-of-pocket spending for health insurance and healthcare has also increased. This increase in out-of-pocket spending has been brought on by higher premiums, deductibles, and copayments for people with health insurance coverage, as well as an overall increase in the number of uninsured people. Between 2000 and 2010, the average premium for family coverage in an employer-provided health insurance plan increased by 114 percent (from $5,438 to $13,770), and the employee's portion of the premium increased by 147 percent (from $1,619 to $3,997) (Claxton et al. 2010). For people who purchase their own health insurance coverage, premiums increased by 18 percent between 2009 and 2010 alone (Kaiser Family Foundation 2010).

The recent economic downturn, coupled with growth in overall healthcare costs and the individual consumer's share of costs, have created significant financial challenges for many households. In a 2008 survey of American families, the Kaiser Family Foundation (2008) reported that 28 percent of people had difficulty paying for healthcare or health insurance. High healthcare spending has a downstream financial effect; 37 percent reported having financial troubles as a result of medical bills. When people must pay healthcare bills, they often have difficulty paying other bills or paying for necessities (e.g., food, housing). They draw down their savings accounts, borrow money, and experience other difficulties. These hardships compel individuals who can't delay treatment to seek high-value care and, as a result, are driving growth in both international and domestic medical travel.

To find high-value care, consumers must be able to compare local options against other alternatives. They need access to reliable information on quality, health outcomes, and price. Without data on all these components, consumers will be unable to find the value they seek.

QUALITY COMPARISONS

For consumers who are seeking the highest-quality providers and willing to travel for care, data are scant and often difficult to interpret. Web-based data sources are improving consumers' access to health data, but they are still in their early stages. Hospital Compare (www .hospitalcompare.hhs.gov), created by the Centers for Medicare & Medicaid Services (CMS), reports quality measures for hospital processes of care (including specific measures related to heart attack, heart failure, pneumonia, surgical care, and pediatric asthma care) and outcomes measures (including 30-day readmission and in-hospital mortality rates by hospital). However, the tool is not designed to identify hospitals with the "best" performance in the nation. Another source of data is Health-Grades, an independent organization that evaluates the quality of healthcare providers, including physicians and hospitals. The HealthGrades website features ratings and comments submitted by patients about their provider experiences (e.g., communication, time spent with physician, ease of scheduling), as well as technical information related to a physician's training, awards, and professional history. It also reports quality-based information gathered by CMS and general cost information (e.g., the amount paid for a procedure or to treat a diagnosis, on average, for a patient with insurance coverage and the "list" price for the treatment, and whether a particular hospital's prices are higher than, the same as, or lower than the state average).

Other high-profile, consumer-oriented rating sites include the *U.S. News and World Report* Best Hospitals site, the Leapfrog Group's site, and Angie's List. The information offered among these and other sites, however, does not appear to match. Research conducted in 2008 found a low level of agreement among four such sites on the rankings of the hospitals studied (Rothberg et al. 2008). Clearly, more work needs to be done to develop quality reporting mechanisms on which consumers can rely when making value-based healthcare decisions.

COST COMPARISONS

Although quality data are limited, they are far more abundant than price data, which are nearly impossible for US consumers to obtain. Often this lack of data stems from providers' inability to quote an inclusive cost for a particular treatment. Hospital and physician services are generally billed separately, and different physicians often generate separate bills. Billing for a hip replacement procedure may include separate bills from the hospital, the orthopedic surgeon, and the anesthesiologist, each from a different billing system. In contrast, for uncomplicated cases, some international providers are able to offer package prices (similar to those offered by the travel industry) that include all fees for the hospital, physician, surgery, lab, medication, and room.

An apples-to-apples comparison of healthcare costs does not encompass the costs associated with travel, however. Travel costs might include air or ground travel to and from the destination and hospital; lodging costs before and after hospitalization, if the patient will be unable to travel immediately following discharge; lodging costs for a companion during hospitalization; food and other incidental costs; and the cost of special travel accommodations (e.g., an economy plus or business class seat during air travel, if the patient needs extra leg room). The opportunity costs associated with medical travel—the value of the patient's and travel companion's time during travel and hospitalization—are also likely to be higher for a number of reasons. The patient and a companion must spend additional time traveling. Hospital lengths of stay can be longer for international patients (Satjapot, Johnson, and Garman 2011). The patient may need to stay near the hospital once discharged for follow-up care, which would also require the companion to extend his stay. Exhibit 4.1 provides an example of differences in travel times and airfares to international medical travel destinations. Airfare and opportunity costs for travel to Monterrey, Mexico, for example, are substantially lower than those for travel to Bangkok, Thailand, or Kuala Lumpur, Malaysia.

These costs would need to be factored into a comprehensive comparison of the costs of care at different destinations. However, comparisons of medical care costs between the United States and international medical travel destinations demonstrate such substantial cost savings that, even after factoring in travel and opportunity costs, medi-cal travel is generally less expensive (see Exhibit 4.2).

WILL CONSUMERS SHOP FOR HIGH-VALUE CARE?

Despite increasing and potentially devastating out-of-pocket healthcare costs, evidence is mixed regarding consumers' willingness to "shop" for high-value care. Milstein and Smith (2007) estimated that only 20–40% of consumers would be willing to travel to a "very good offshore hospital with very good physicians" if they saved at least $10,000. Other research suggests that consumers are skeptical about the notions of cost savings in healthcare and shopping around for high-value care. For example, a 2010 study found that consumers perceived more care to be higher-quality care, newer technologies to be better technologies, and more costly care to be better care (Carman et al. 2010). The results of this study suggest that the average US consumer will need to overcome a number of misperceptions to believe that high-quality care can be lower cost. Furthermore, without comparable quality information, transparency of cost information as a mechanism to motivate value-based purchasing could ultimately backfire.

EXHIBIT 4.1: Examples of Travel Distances and Prices (US$) from Major US Cities to International Medical Travel Destinations

	Chicago		Los Angeles		Miami	
	Distance	Price	Distance	Price	Distance	Price
Bogota, Colombia	7'17"	$316	8'42"	$590	3'25"	$299
San Jose, Costa Rica	6'45"	$423	5'50"	$559	2'45"	$333
New Delhi, India	14'30"	$1,264	19'45"	$1,390	18'00"	$1,313
Amman, Jordan	12'00"	$1,307	19'58"	$4,503	18'16"	$1,626
Seoul, Korea	13'35"	$1,170	12'55"	$1,301	17'36"	$1,758
Monterrey, Mexico	3'25"	$737	5'35"	$642	3'00"	$521
Tel Aviv, Israel	14'00"	$1,602	17'00"	$4,229	14'30"	$5,481
Bangkok, Thailand	19'46"	$3,617	17'20"	$1,369	24'11"	$3,509
Ho Chi Min City, Vietnam	21'15"	$4,105	17'55"	$1,109	24'20"	$4,368
Kuala Lumpur, Malaysia	22'25"	$2,603	19'45"	$1,279	22'55"	$3,804
Managua, Nicaragua	6'55"	$376	6'57"	$578	2'35"	$346

SOURCE: Author calculations based on flights retrieved from www.travelocity.com on July 22, 2010.

THE EVOLUTION OF MEDICAL TRAVEL: FROM LONG-HAUL TO SHORT-HAUL DESTINATIONS

Some of the first medical tourism providers to advertise to Americans were located in "long-haul" destinations—destinations that took seven hours or more to reach via nonstop flight. Even without medical treatment, long-haul travel can be exhausting, requiring up to 24 hours or more travel time. For this reason

EXHIBIT 4.2: Comparison of Medical Care Costs Across Countries, in Thousands (US$)

	USA	Colombia	Costa Rica	India	Jordan	Korea	Mexico	Israel	Thailand	Vietnam	Malaysia	Nicaragua
Heart bypass	144.0	14.8	25.0	5.2	14.4	28.9	27.0	27.5	15.1	NA	11.4	NA
Angioplasty	57.0	4.5	13.0	3.3	5.0	15.2	12.5	8.0	3.8	NA	5.4	NA
Heart valve replacement	170.0	18.0	30.0	5.5	14.4	43.5	18.0	29.7	21.2	NA	10.6	NA
Hip replacement	50.0	6.5	12.5	7.0	8.0	14.1	13.0	25.3	7.9	8.3	7.5	8.7
Hip resurfacing	50.0	10.5	12.5	7.0	10.0	15.6	15.0	20.0	15.2	NA	12.4	NA
Knee replacement	50.0	6.5	11.5	6.2	8.0	19.8	12.0	24.9	12.3	8.5	7.0	8.2
Spinal fusion	100.0	NA	11.5	6.5	10.0	15.4	12.0	35.0	9.1	6.2	6.0	NA
Dental implant	2.8	1.8	0.9	1.0	1.0	4.2	1.8	2.2	3.6	NA	0.4	NA
Gastric sleeve	28.7	7.2	10.5	5.0	NA	NA	10.0	11.5	13.6	NA	NA	8.0
Gastric bypass	32.9	9.9	12.5	5.0	NA	NA	11.0	11.5	16.7	NA	9.5	8.0
Lap band	30.0	9.9	8.5	3.0	7.0	NA	6.5	1.0	11.5	NA	NA	8.0
Liposuction	9.0	2.5	3.9	2.8	4.0	NA	2.8	7.2	2.3	2.9	2.3	NA
Tummy tuck	9.8	3.5	5.3	3.0	4.0	NA	4.0	11.0	5.0	3.9	NA	NA
Breast implants	10.0	2.5	3.8	3.5	3.5	12.5	3.5	21.0	2.7	3.9	NA	4.4
Rhinoplasty	8.0	2.5	4.5	4.0	3.0	5.0	3.5	9.5	3.1	2.1	1.3	2.4
Face lift	15.0	5.0	6.0	4.0	4.4	15.3	4.9	16.0	3.7	4.2	3.4	NA
Hysterectomy	15.0	NA	5.7	2.5	6.0	11.0	5.8	14.0	2.7	NA	5.3	3.0
Lasik (both eyes)	4.4	2.0	1.8	0.5	5.0	6.0	2.0	NA	1.8	1.6	0.5	NA
IVF treatments	14.5	NA	2.8	3.3	2.7	2.2	4.0	2.8	9.1	NA	3.8	NA

SOURCE: Data from Medical Tourism Association (2010).
NOTES: Prices do not reflect PPO discounts; prices will vary on the basis of zip code, region, provider, and other factors.

alone, long-haul destinations, such as Thailand, Singapore, and India, are likely to remain a relatively small proportion of total medical care (see Exhibit 4.3).

More recently, countries closer to the United States have become medical travel destinations for Americans. Costa Rica, Mexico, Panama, and Nicaragua are advertising medical care that requires a quarter of the time needed to travel to long-haul destinations. While the costs of medical care at the short-haul destinations might be higher than the costs of care at farther destinations, lower travel and opportunity costs could offset the higher medical costs.

The latest evolution of medical travel is domestic medical travel. Galichia Hospital in Wichita, Kansas, for example, markets itself as a heart hospital caring for medical travelers, offering cardiac and heart bypass surgery at an all-inclusive price of $12,000 regardless of hospital length of stay (www.galichiamedicaltourism .com). Some health insurers, such as BridgeHealth, now offer national networks of providers, thereby facilitating domestic medical travel. These insurers may also contract for

EXHIBIT 4.3: Evolution of Medical Travel

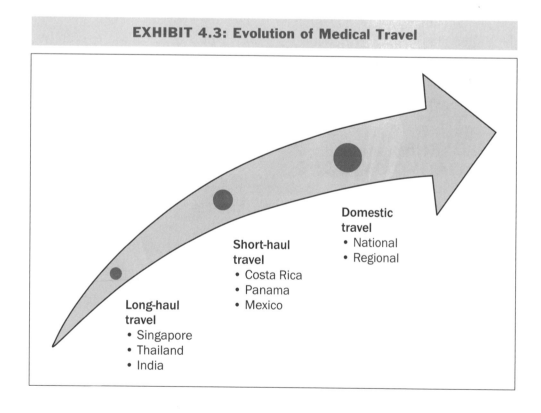

Domestic travel
• National
• Regional

Short-haul travel
• Costa Rica
• Panama
• Mexico

Long-haul travel
• Singapore
• Thailand
• India

inclusive pricing of hospital and physician care rather than for traditional "piecemeal" pricing. Hospitals and physicians have traditionally been paid separately; a flat diagnosis-related group (DRG) payment is made to the hospital for the hospital stay, and separate payments based on a negotiated fee schedule are made for each service provided by a physician. The traditional fragmented payment system often translates into higher costs than a patient or insurer projected, due to the inability of the hospital and physicians to provide a single estimate of the cost of care. With greater price transparency and competition among providers within the United States, a shift toward all-inclusive pricing for treatments may facilitate and encourage more domestic medical travel.

EMPLOYERS NEGOTIATING ON VALUE

With skyrocketing healthcare costs, employers have a strong impetus to negotiate contractual arrangements that provide the highest-value care for their employees, which could mean incentivizing employees to travel domestically or abroad to high-value providers. Self-insured employers, which act as their own insurance

company to provide health insurance to their employees, have a direct incentive to reduce healthcare costs by contracting with low-cost, high-value providers.

Employers have begun to negotiate more aggressively on value with international and domestic providers. In 2007 Hannaford Bros. in Maine became one of the first employers to negotiate a contract with a provider outside of the United States for certain surgeries in an effort to reduce costs without compromising coverage or quality. In response to the potential loss of patients to providers abroad, local providers negotiated lower rates with the company (Appleby 2010). More recently, both employers and intermediaries have begun to strategically negotiate with domestic providers that perform well on quality measures if they are willing to accept lower reimbursement in exchange for the potential to treat larger numbers of patients. In February 2010, Lowe's, a national home improvement retail chain, announced a contract with Cleveland Clinic to provide cardiac procedures to its 228,000 employees and their dependents as a national alternative to local providers. While the plan did not require enrollees to seek care from Cleveland Clinic, it offered financial incentives, such as deductible waivers and reimbursement of travel costs for the patient and a companion, to encourage travel to Cleveland Clinic (Appleby 2010; Cleveland Clinic 2010).

WHAT DO THESE TRENDS MEAN FOR THE FUTURE?

The activities described in this chapter are just the tip of the iceberg for regional and national competition. The Patient Protection and Affordable Care Act (P.L. 111-148) will fund a private, nonprofit institute to conduct patient-centered outcomes research; develop a "Physician Compare" website, similar to CMS's Hospital Compare website, to provide quality-related information about doctors; and create a methodology for measuring health plan value. When more rigorous and systematic comparisons of health outcomes and risks, benefits, and clinical effectiveness of different medical treatments become available, con-

sumers will have the tools they need to make better value-based decisions about treatment alternatives. At the same time, consumers need rigorous comparative quality and performance data on physicians and hospitals so they can make decisions not only about treatment options but also about the providers that will provide the treatment. These two developments, taken together, will significantly improve the consumer's ability to accurately assess quality.

As better quality data continue to be developed and competition from international providers continues to grow, US providers will need to improve their price transparency. Competition for patients, which has historically been a local phenomenon, will increase at the regional and national level for procedures that can be scheduled in advance. Both employers and insurers will more actively search for the highest-value healthcare and turn to domestic medical travel as a strategy to reduce long-term healthcare costs.

CHAPTER 5

The Changing Nature of Healthcare Demand in a Global Context

The American public's main concern about healthcare is cost. Healthcare expenditures in the United States are the highest in the world, averaging $7,358 per person in 2008, compared to $3,060 (adjusted for purchasing power) in other member countries of the Organisation of Economic Co-operation and Development (OECD 2010a). OECD is an economic organization comprising 33 democratic, market-based member countries that focuses on improving economic and social welfare. The United States spent almost 50 percent more on healthcare than Norway ($5,003 per capita) and Switzerland ($4,627 per capita), which ranked second and third among the OECD's highest spenders (OECD 2010a). Healthcare spending as a proportion of gross domestic product (GDP) has increased by 3.4 percent annually between 2000 and 2008, far outpacing the 1.2 percent annual growth in GDP overall (see Exhibit 5.1). However, these statistics do not tell the whole story about how healthcare spending in the United States compares to healthcare spending in other countries.

As fast as our costs are growing, two-thirds of the other OECD countries' costs are growing even faster. Between 2000 and 2008, Slovakia's annual spending grew the fastest, at a rate of 11.0 percent. More notably, several countries that are often compared to the United States had higher annual growth rates, including New Zealand (4.7 percent), the United Kingdom (4.6 percent), The Netherlands (4.3 percent), Denmark (3.7 percent), and Sweden (3.6 percent). Furthermore, while annual healthcare spending increased three times as fast as GDP in the United States, healthcare spending increased six times as fast as GDP in Portugal and five times as fast in Italy. In other words, we are not the only country facing an unsustainable cost curve.

In the United States, much of the focus on "bending the cost curve" has been on service costs—the supply side of the equation. While improving the efficiency with which care is provided is an important part of reducing healthcare costs, in the context of increasing demand it will not provide a complete solution. In this chapter, we consider five important demand-related trends affecting healthcare delivery systems in the United States and other countries and the effect these trends will have on us in the future.

THE CHANGING COMPOSITION OF THE US POPULATION

The US population is expected to grow by 20 percent between 2010 and 2030, adding 63.2 million people (see Exhibit 5.2) (US Census Bureau 2008). More important, the number of people aged 65 to 84 will grow by 28.9 million (84 percent). The number of the "oldest old" (people aged 85 or older) will grow by only 3 million (52 percent); however, this group has a disproportionately large number of people with multiple complex health and social support needs.

Although growth in annual healthcare spending in the United States has been dramatic . . .

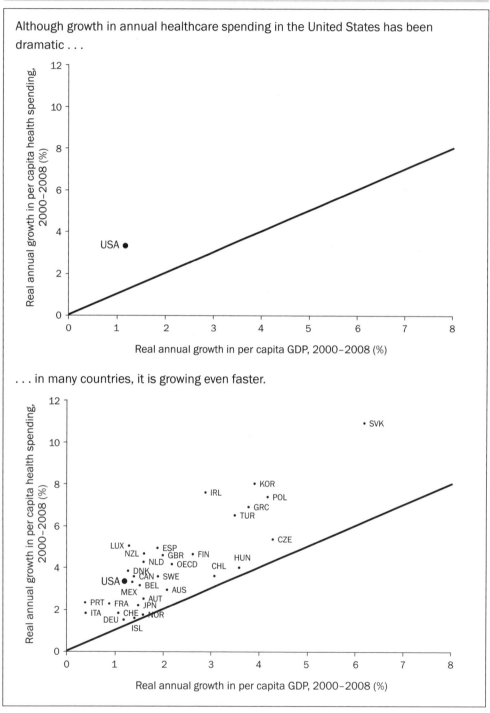

. . . in many countries, it is growing even faster.

SOURCE: Data from OECD (2010c).
NOTES: Data for Luxembourg and Portugal are for years 2000–2006; for Australia, Denmark, Greece, Japan, and Turkey, 2000–2007; and for Iceland, 2000–2009.

EXHIBIT 5.2: Population Growth, 2010–2030 by Age, in Thousands

	2010	**2030**	**Absolute Change**	**% Change**
Overall	310,233	373,504	63,271	20.4
Age group				
<18 years	75,217	87,815	12,598	16.7
18–24	30,713	34,059	3,346	10.9
25–44	83,095	95,242	12,147	14.6
45–64	80,980	84,296	3,316	4.1
65–84	34,478	63,347	28,869	83.7
85 or older	5,751	8,745	2,994	52.1

SOURCE: Author calculations based on data from US Census Bureau (2008).

Although these trends are likely to require us to make substantial adjustments, we will not need to be at the vanguard of these solutions. That burden falls on Japan, the country with the oldest population. Twenty-two percent of Japan's population is aged 65 or older, compared to just 13 percent in the United States (Arai 2009; US Census Bureau 2008). The populations of Italy and Germany closely follow Japan, both at 20 percent (OECD 2010b).

What can the United States learn from these countries? Two common strategies have emerged: public sector funding of long-term care and support of healthy aging at home.

The majority of care for older adults in Germany and Japan is provided at home and combines formal and informal care (Rechel et al. 2009; Campbell, Ikegami, and Gibson 2010). Both countries have publicly funded long-term care insurance programs to address coverage and equity for older adults. Unlike the United States, where more than two-thirds of public funding for long-term care is spent on nursing homes, Germany and Japan spend considerably more on helping people live at home successfully as long as possible. To this end, Germany offers a cash allowance and direct service provision, including care at home (e.g., home help) and some limited care outside the home (e.g., night care, short stays in nursing homes), to older adults; consumers can use either or both. Japan funds only direct provision of services.

Informal caregiving plays an important role in providing social and familial support for older adults. In addition, given the growth in the number of older adults needing care at home, the supply of formal caregivers would likely be insufficient to meet the demand for care if all care were provided formally. A common criticism of formal care is that it may substitute for, rather than enhance, informal caregiving; however, research suggests that they are complements and, when used together, expand the services available to older adults (Rechel et al. 2009). Both cash allowances and direct service provision are viewed as means to use public monies for

supplementing, rather than replacing, informal care (Campbell, Ikegami, and Gibson 2010).

European countries also provide an infrastructure, social support services, and low-tech, holistic, nonmedical strategies to keep older people living at home longer. Because most of the care of older people is provided in the home, in larger communities resources are generally located nearby, and basic needs such as food and household goods can be purchased from shops in proximity. The public transportation infrastructure in many European cities provides older adults with easy access to transit, with many bus/ train stops located within walking distance of home.

INCREASING EXPERIENCES ABROAD

Growth of the Internet has made it easier to learn about tourism in other countries and to search for low fares between the United States and destinations abroad and has led to a steady increase in international travel since the 1990s. The number of flights taken abroad by US residents increased by 52 percent between 1995 and 2009, while the number of inbound flights taken by non-US residents from other countries increased by only 15 percent in that same period (Exhibit 5.3) (US Department of Commerce, International Trade Administration Office of Travel & Tourism Industries 2010).

In addition, more young Americans are studying abroad during college and experiencing different cultural, social, and healthcare systems that may ultimately shape their lifetime perceptions and expectations about the US healthcare system. Between the 1995–1996 and 2007–2008 academic years, the number of college students studying abroad increased by nearly 200 percent, from 89,242 to 262,416

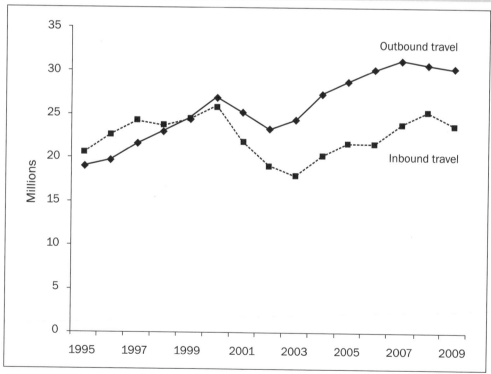

EXHIBIT 5.3: Number of Inbound and Outbound Air Travelers, 1995–2009

SOURCE: US Department of Commerce, International Trade Administration Office of Travel & Tourism Industries (2010).
NOTE: Chart reflects overseas flights only; travel to Canada and Mexico is excluded.

(IIE Network 2009). This increase demonstrates an interest in living and working in a global environment. Along with international experience, they are gaining a greater understanding of what works in other systems, and healthcare is no exception. Many European systems, for example, are predicated on the principle of *solidarity*, the unity of a community or group grounded in shared interests, mutual support, and reciprocity. In an economic context, it can also refer to the provision of public goods to all members of a society (Hartwig and Nicolaides 2003). Through exposure to different healthcare systems, students abroad experience firsthand how different systems address morbidity and mortality-related health problems at a lower cost and with similar or better outcomes. This group's greater appreciation for solidarity, common interests, and expectations could influence public opinion concerning future health reform.

CONTINUED GROWTH IN "LIFESTYLE" DISEASES

The number of people with lifestyle-related chronic diseases, such as diabetes, heart disease, stroke, high blood pressure, and some cancers,

will continue to increase over the coming years due to unhealthy diet and poor nutrition, sedentary lifestyles, and smoking, in addition to the aging of the population. The burden of chronic disease is insidious, affecting quality of life, healthcare costs, and employer costs (through lost productivity). Growth of lifestyle diseases will outpace population growth in the near future. Between 2003 and 2023, the proportion of Americans with diabetes is projected to increase by 53 percent; with heart disease, by 41 percent; with hypertension, by 39 percent; and affected by stroke, by 29 percent, while the population is projected to increase by 19 percent overall (see Exhibit 5.4) (Bodenheimer, Chen, and Bennett 2009).

What can we do to change lifestyles and ultimately slow the growth of chronic disease? Medical care has become the primary strategy for improving health in the United States; behaviorally and environmentally grounded approaches receive less attention here than in other countries. Tremendous resources have been spent on medical innovations to treat or cure disease, but more resources could be invested in developing and testing less invasive nonmedical strategies to prevent disease and

EXHIBIT 5.4: Comparing the Increases in Total Costs Associated with Chronic Conditions

Chronic Disease	Increase in Prevalence, 2003–2023	Increase in Total Costs, 2003–2023
Overall chronic illness	42%	$2.9 trillion
Diabetes	53%	$298 billion
Hypertension	39%	$615 billion
Heart disease	41%	$758 billion
Stroke	29%	$62 billion

SOURCE: Data from Bodenheimer, Chen, and Bennett (2009).
NOTES: The overall population will grow by 19 percent between 2003 and 2023; total costs include healthcare and on-the-job productivity losses; overall chronic illness includes costs incurred as a result of cancers, diabetes, hypertension, stroke, heart disease, pulmonary conditions, and mental disorders.

improve overall health. For example, while sedentary lifestyle is a risk factor associated with obesity, hypertension, and heart disease, we have put few practices into place that motivate people to become and remain physically active.

CONTINUED GROWTH IN MEDICAL TECHNOLOGY

Medical technologies—the procedures, drugs, equipment, devices, and processes used to provide

medical care—are another important factor stimulating demand. Technologies targeting previously untreatable conditions increase the demand for medical care by increasing the number of people who seek treatment. Technologies can also have a "substitution effect," shifting demand away from existing treatments. For example, minimally invasive hip replacement has shifted demand away from traditional hip replacement procedures. To the extent that the substitute technologies improve the process, value, or outcomes of care, they can also generate new demand. In the example of hip replacement, the development of minimally invasive procedures has created new demand by people who would otherwise forgo treatment due to concerns about recovery time.

New medical technologies accounted for 27 to 48 percent of the growth in healthcare spending between 1960 and 2007 (Smith, Newhouse, and Freeland 2009). However, future growth in new technologies brought to the US market may be tempered by new regulations. The Patient Protection and Affordable Care Act levies a 2.3 percent excise tax on medical devices, which could stem innovation, particularly innovation by small medical device companies and start-ups, in coming years (Nexon and Ubl 2010). While a portion of the tax will ultimately be passed onto the consumer, the proportion of the tax that will be borne by the consumer versus the medical device companies is not yet clear, and the extent to which the excise tax will slow the introduction of new devices is yet to be seen.

What does new technology mean for US healthcare providers and the system more generally? Currently, the introduction of new technologies is not restricted by value, relative to existing technologies in the United States. Although the typical US consumer believes that newer technologies are superior to existing technologies and more expensive treatments are better (Carman et al. 2010), in reality some new technologies improve quality or outcomes or decrease costs, while others neither improve quality or outcomes nor decrease costs relative to existing technologies. To fully implement evidence-based medicine and provide the highest quality of care possible, new technologies will need to deliver improvements in value. One of the first systematic efforts toward this goal in the United States was the American Recovery and Reinvestment Act of 2009, which supported the development of a comparative effectiveness research program by the National Institutes of Health.

While comparison of effectiveness is a crucial step in identifying high-value care, the next logical step is to systematically examine the cost-effectiveness of alternative treatments. Here, too, we can benefit from the progress and lessons learned from other countries that have pioneered these efforts. We will return to this topic in Chapter 8.

GROWING INCOME INEQUALITIES

In the United States, there has been a growing trend toward income inequality—i.e., the difference between what people in the top and bottom of the income range earn. Income growth for households earning in the 95th percentile has consistently outpaced income growth for lower-earning households, widening the gap between the highest and lowest income earners (see Exhibit 5.5) (DeNavas-Walt, Proctor, and Smith, US Census Bureau 2010). This income inequality has grown 21 percent between 1968 and 2008, putting us in the top third of all countries when ranked from lowest to highest income inequality (see Exhibit 5.6). The US level of inequality is more typical of developing countries; the only developed countries with higher income inequality are Hong Kong and Singapore (Central Intelligence Agency 2010).

These income inequalities are also associated with large health disparities. Most developed countries have relatively egalitarian distributions of income compared to the United States, and their social insurance systems are predicated on solidarity, or a "we-feeling." A foundation in solidarity supports universal coverage and equal access throughout a nation. Although the healthcare reform passed in 2010 takes an important step toward universal coverage, without a commensurate change in economic inequity, disparities in access and quality are likely to persist.

SUMMARY

The United States and countries across the world need sustainable solutions to the cost curve problem. While the United States faces challenges that other developed countries do not, the nation stands to learn from their success in facing similar problems. In some instances, other countries have come up with innovative solutions that address the challenges; in other cases, we are at similar points.

Opportunities to learn and benefit from each other are likely to expand in the future as a result of another macro trend we will consider in Chapter 7: convergence and harmonization across borders.

Income growth for households in the 95th percentile has consistently outpaced income growth for lower-earning households . . .

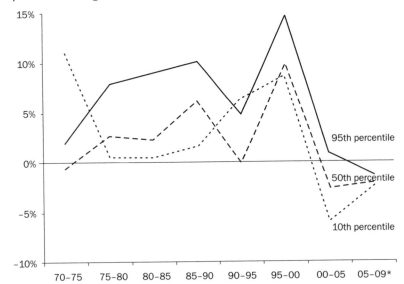

. . . resulting in a growing disparity between the highest- and lowest-earning households.

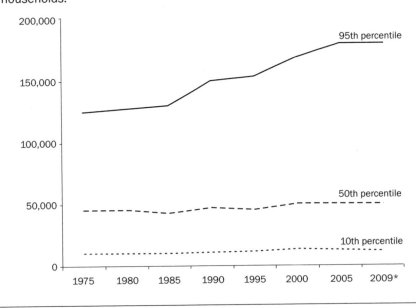

SOURCE: Data from DeNavas-Walt, Proctor, and Smith, US Census Bureau (2010).
*2009 is the most recent year of data available.

EXHIBIT 5.6: Growing Income Inequality in the United States Compared to Other Countries

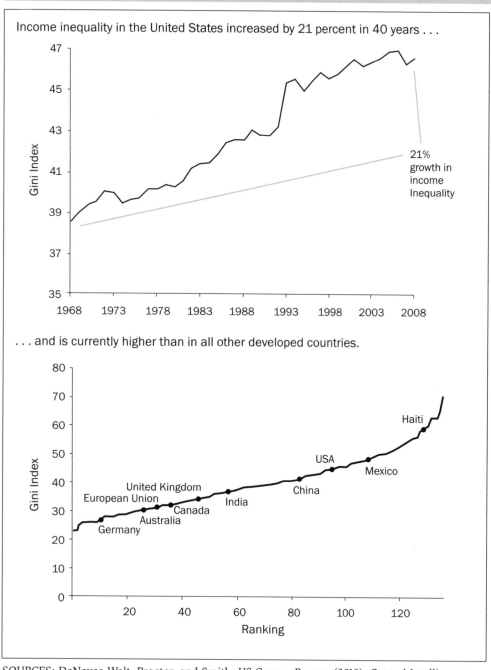

Income inequality in the United States increased by 21 percent in 40 years . . .

. . . and is currently higher than in all other developed countries.

SOURCES: DeNavas-Walt, Proctor, and Smith, US Census Bureau (2010); Central Intelligence Agency (2010).

CHAPTER 6

The Growing Mobility of Health Professionals

Several years ago, a colleague in Singapore described his nation-state's healthcare workforce challenges to me (AG). Like most other countries' hospitals, Singapore's hospitals were facing shortages of healthcare professionals—nursing personnel in particular. To address the need for more physicians, the Ministry of Health liberalized its credentialing of internationally trained doctors. In nursing, Singapore was able to find a particularly innovative niche that helped it build a pipeline. It had observed that skilled nurses were drawn to Singapore from other countries for the higher wages they could receive there; once they had learned English, however, they would leave to pursue still higher wages in the United States. Rather than trying to prevent this trend, Singapore embraced it. It built a marketing campaign around the opportunity to practice in Singapore and learn English and even offered to help nurses seeking to make a temporary stop there on their journey to the United States.

This example is a microcosm of global trends toward greater cross-border mobility of health professionals. Historically, this migration has benefitted the United States. Global comparisons consistently show that the United States provides the highest incomes for nurses and general practitioners and among the highest incomes for specialists (Fujisawa and Lafortune 2007; Peterson and Burton 2007), making it a prime destination for health professionals. In the future, this trend may start to tip in the other direction.

TRENDS IN PROFESSIONAL MIGRATION

The American Association of Medical Colleges' Center for Workforce Studies has projected that the United States will face a shortage of 159,000 physicians by 2025 (Dill and Salsberg 2008). The shortfall is more pronounced when we look at the need for primary care physicians, particularly in underserved areas. A trend toward outward migration of physicians from the United States could make these shortfalls even more severe.

The number of international medical graduates (IMGs)—physicians who received their training outside the United States and Canada—has been growing since 1981. Today IMGs account for more than 25 percent of the physician workforce across the United States (American Medical Association 2010). Exhibit 6.1 compares GDP growth in the United States to growth in the five countries in which the largest numbers of IMGs completed their training. Cumulatively these five countries represent about 43 percent of the total IMG workforce in the United States. Growth has slowed across the globe during this period, as shown in the top half of the exhibit, and if we stopped there we might take comfort in all the company we have. If we look at the *cumulative* growth since 2007 shown in the bottom half of the exhibit,

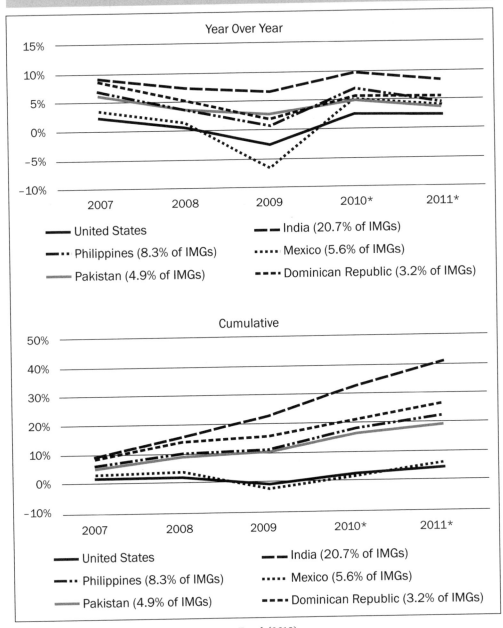

EXHIBIT 6.1: GDP Growth Rate, 2007–2009, United States Versus Its Top Five Sources of IMGs

Year Over Year

— United States

— — India (20.7% of IMGs)

—·· Philippines (8.3% of IMGs)

····· Mexico (5.6% of IMGs)

— Pakistan (4.9% of IMGs)

—–·· Dominican Republic (3.2% of IMGs)

Cumulative

— United States

— — India (20.7% of IMGs)

—·· Philippines (8.3% of IMGs)

····· Mexico (5.6% of IMGs)

— Pakistan (4.9% of IMGs)

—–·· Dominican Republic (3.2% of IMGs)

SOURCE: Data from International Monetary Fund (2010).
*Estimated

however, a different picture emerges. Here we more clearly see that the dominant trend is the increasing strength of these source countries' economies. With stronger economies come higher demands for services such as healthcare, as well as for the resources needed to support those services.

DEMAND AND SUPPLY SHOCKS

A *shock* is a sudden change in demand or supply. In terms of workforce, shocks can be created by a variety of sources. Legislated changes in working hours and conditions (e.g., nurse-to-patient ratios) are familiar sources of shocks in the United States. Shocks can also come from the introduction of new technologies, catastrophic environmental events, and immigration pattern shifts caused by favorable or unfavorable changes in a given region (OECD 2008).

Let's return to the example of the developing economies in countries that historically contributed doctors to the United States. Imagine that a country wants to substantially expand its domestic healthcare and decides to expand both its hospitals and its education programs. New hospitals may take 3 to 5 years to build from plan to opening, but it takes 11 years or more to educate and train a new doctor. Thus, the country has two choices: It can delay opening new hospitals for 6 to 8 years post-construction while the new doctors complete their education, or it can find the doctors it needs from other regions. Many clinicians came to the United States for the greater opportunities they could find here, but when similar opportunities emerge in their home countries, how many can we count on to stay here? As these home economies continue to emerge, we need to proactively address their potential impact on the IMG population.

CHAPTER 7

Convergence and Harmonization

Once CHRISTUS Health expanded into Mexico, it quickly identified opportunities to improve value in its facilities. One opportunity involved developing local partnerships for the production of minor healthcare supplies, such as bandages and intravenous drips. Because labor and other costs were lower in Mexico, local manufacturers would be able to produce supplies at a level of quality comparable to that in the United States at 50 to 60 percent of the cost. To ensure comparable quality standards were developed and maintained, CHRISTUS pursued these opportunities through joint venture. This arrangement benefited the patient because it drove down costs without compromising quality, and local communities benefited from the additional economic activity these manufacturers provided.

The experience of CHRISTUS Health is just one example of a company taking innovative approaches to meeting healthcare needs in lower-income areas. The size of the healthcare market in emerging economies, an estimated $200 billion, has also drawn the attention of larger companies, such as Procter & Gamble and General Electric, that are pursuing strategies to "reverse engineer" products from the developed world to work within the economic constraints of the developing world (Byron 2007; Hammond et al. 2007; Immelt, Govindarajan, and Trimble 2009).

All of the above begs the question: If these products can be made more efficient, or more efficiently, couldn't these new approaches also help the developed world as we strive to control our own escalating costs? They could, but there are considerable barriers to entering developed markets, many having to do with regulatory systems that do not lend themselves to cross-border strategies.

HEALTHCARE: LOCAL BY DESIGN

Two substantial challenges in adapting knowledge and innovations from other countries are (1) the disparate regulations covering healthcare, health insurance, patents, and new technologies and (2) the different, and sometimes conflicting, standards and practices among organizations. "Hard" cross-country or cross-jurisdiction borders inhibit the transfer of innovation, but greater cooperation among countries to diffuse innovations could increase efficiency and the speed of adoption. Convergence occurs when laws, regulations, or practices across companies, states, countries, or other jurisdictions become more similar or standardized, regardless of whether the growing similarities are planned or unplanned. Harmonization is a type of convergence, where the laws, regulations, or practices become more similar in a planful way, to address inconsistencies and interdependence among parties. Convergence, and harmonization in particular, can improve efficiency in disseminating innovations and best practices. What are some opportunities for greater harmonization within the United

States and among the United States and other countries?

PRICE TRANSPARENCY

We have described price and quality transparency in previous chapters. In the era of consumer-driven healthcare, consumers are encouraged to participate more actively in their healthcare decisions. To do so, they need access to information they can understand and use to directly compare their options. Some of the largest providers abroad catering to American patients advertise average prices for different treatments and will provide firm quotes if requested. As more international providers publish all-inclusive prices for medical and surgical treatments, competition from abroad could facilitate domestic price transparency in a few US markets. Greater price transparency in even a few domestic markets could ultimately be a tipping point toward price transparency across the rest of the United States. As has been seen in other industries, such as the airline industry, harmonization of price transparency would encourage more competition domestically and internationally. Nathan Cortez (2009), assistant professor in the Dedman School of Law at Southern Methodist University, coined the term *market-driven convergence* to describe harmonization instigated by private sector needs for more uniform standards and practices.

QUALITY AND ACCREDITATION

Hospital quality accreditation is an example of an area in which healthcare has begun to converge internationally. Joint Commission International (JCI) accreditation is widely viewed as the "gold standard" of quality for hospitals that cater to international patients. JCI accreditation is voluntary, but the number of JCI-accredited hospitals worldwide has grown more than twentyfold since 2002 (see Exhibit 7.1). Having seen hospitals that serve international patients use their JCI accreditation as a marketing tool to attract patients, other hospitals have quickly followed suit.

PROVIDER PAYMENT INCENTIVES

Within the United States, the healthcare system could gain efficiency by aligning provider payment incentives across payers. In the current system, a single provider receives payments

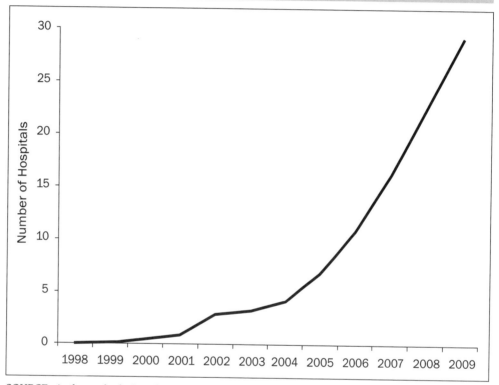

EXHIBIT 7.1: Growth in Number of Hospitals with Joint Commission International Accreditation

SOURCE: Author calculations based on register of accredited organizations at Joint Commission International (2010).

based on a variety of arrangements, such as per diem rates, capitation, and fee-for-service. These payment methodologies carry different and often conflicting incentives. Harmonization of payment schemes to incentivize high-value care could ultimately change how care is delivered. Medicare's Physician Quality Reporting Initiative (PQRI) is one example of how payers are incentivizing quality. For an individual provider, however, PQRI incentive payments may represent a minute portion of his overall revenue because the measures apply only to Medicare patients. For many physicians, the PQRI financial incentive to change their behavior is weak. If private and public payers harmonized their payment methodologies and quality incentives, a greater portion of revenue (or costs) would be at stake, and this prospect would be a more powerful influence on behavior. Private payers often follow Medicare's lead, but metrics and targets nevertheless differ among private and public payers.

With the passing of the Patient Protection and Affordable Care Act of 2010, coordination of care may converge on accountable care organizations (ACOs). ACOs are designed to better align payments with coordination of care and quality by shifting risk to providers for the overall care provided to individual patients through financial incentives. However, financial incentives for ACO providers can vary substantially, from low-risk arrangements that use fee-for-service payments coupled with shared savings or bonuses for meeting quality targets to high-risk arrangements that rely on capitation and bundled payments (Shortell, Casalino, and Fisher 2010). If ACOs are shown to be successful at improving quality, further convergence on a smaller set of financial incentives that change behavior may occur.

LOOKING TO OTHER COUNTRIES AS A SOURCE OF COST INNOVATION

Historically, the United States has rarely looked to other developed countries, and even more rarely to emerging countries, for solutions to its healthcare problems. A common explanation for this provincial orientation is that the US healthcare system is market based, and reliance on the market for health insurance and healthcare makes translation of payment, process, and system innovations to the United States difficult. Although private health insurance plays a more predominant role in the United States than in other developed countries, public health insurance also plays a dominant role. Public insurers, primarily Medicare and Medicaid, covered nearly half (46 percent) of healthcare expenditures in 2008. Other developed countries use a combination of public and private insurance coverage. Some countries that rely heavily on private insurance coverage include South Korea, Switzerland, Greece, and Australia (see Exhibit 7.2) (OECD 2010a). With challenges including insufficient public health infrastructure, inadequate supply of primary

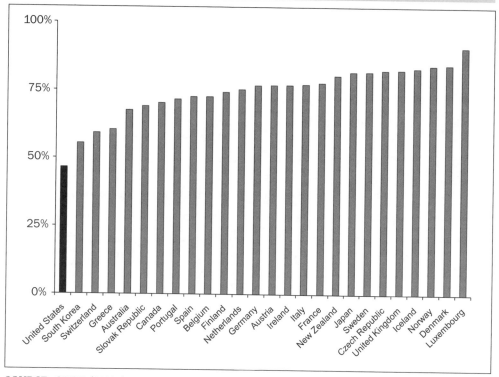

EXHIBIT 7.2: Public Health Expenditures as a Proportion of Total Health Expenditures Per Capita, 2008

SOURCE: OECD (2010a).

care and specialty physicians, and underdeveloped public and private health insurance systems, emerging countries historically have not been perceived as dominant developers of innovations that are relevant to the United States.

This status quo has been changing across industries, and healthcare is not an exception. Developed and emerging countries alike are developing innovative, low-cost solutions that address some of the same problems the US healthcare industry is facing. Emerging markets are now a new source of innovation for the United States in its struggle to fill the gap between how care is currently delivered and the demand for cost-conscious, "frugal" care as a means of slowing healthcare spending (Wooldridge 2010).

As we discussed in Chapter 5, new technologies are a major contributor to increasing healthcare costs in the United States. One strategy the United States could use to bend the cost curve would be to strategically bring high-value technologies to the US market. By reducing costs for the research and development of high-value technologies, we could slow the growth in healthcare spending even more. Clinical trials for new drugs and biologics reviewed by the Federal Drug Administration (FDA) already rely on both domestic and foreign data. In 2008, 86 percent of drug and biologic applications included foreign data (e.g., clinical trials conducted in other countries) and 78 percent of clinical trial subjects were enrolled in sites outside the United States. The proportion of clinical investigators who are outside of the United States has doubled since 1998, and this trend is anticipated to continue, suggesting that the number of foreign clinical trials will also continue to grow (US Department of Health and Human Services, Office of Inspector General 2010).

As clinical trials for new technologies become more global, regulations and data requirements may begin to converge, ultimately reducing unnecessary duplication of research and development and transaction costs (e.g., the costs of submitting a marketing application for a new drug to the FDA). Another systematic effort to harmonize drug development and regulatory approval is the International Conference on Harmonisation of Technical Requirements for Registration of Pharmaceuticals for Human Use (ICH), a collaboration between the United States, Japan, and Europe, whose purpose is to reduce the duplicative testing that is requisite to research and development and to bringing new products to market in different countries (Cortez 2009; ICH 2000).

WHAT'S NEXT?

Harmonization can enable innovation, but it can also stifle it in several ways. If emerging countries try to adopt practices and standards from developed countries, for example, these countries may shift resources to retrofit existing technologies, away from innovative, from-the-ground-up engineering of new high-value solutions. Because harmonization consciously standardizes practices or policies, some may adopt the practice or policy simply because it is "tried and true" rather than rigorously evaluate whether it will work within their political, social, financial, and organizational structures.

Exhibit 7.3 illustrates the cycle of innovation and market convergence—how convergence on a practice, standard, or policy can lead to future innovations. Medical travel is an example of this cycle. Convergence across many countries on medical standards and practices for common procedures (e.g., heart bypass surgery, joint replacements) has made it easier for value-conscious patients to search for and select providers abroad and as a result has prompted more people to travel outside of their home region for medical care. Domestic providers are experiencing increased competition outside the United States as a result of increased accessibility to providers abroad. Increased competition, in turn, has led to the growth of private insurance products that specifically

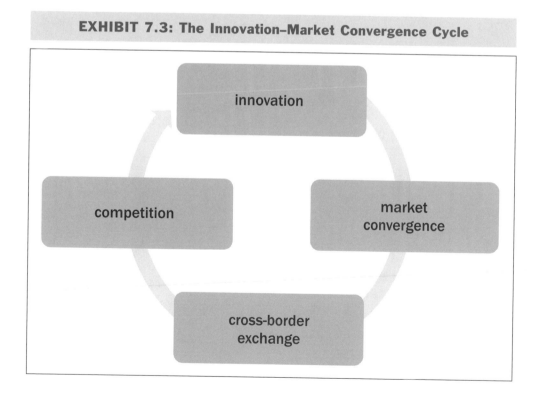

EXHIBIT 7.3: The Innovation–Market Convergence Cycle

address the demands of patients wanting to travel to another country for care. Examples of insurance products designed to cover enrollees in the United States and Mexico include SIMNSA (www.simnsa.org) and Blue Shield of California's Access Baja HMO (www.blueshieldca.com), which provide cross-border health insurance coverage for US employers and their employees in the United States and Mexico.

In this chapter, we have focused on the convergence of practices and standards that has occurred primarily as a result of market-based efforts and on the future of healthcare as states, countries, and other jurisdictions become more similar. In the final chapter, we describe national efforts to standardize the assessment of new technology. We examine different models of assessment and how government payers in other countries systematically evaluate effectiveness and efficiency to identify high-value care when making coverage and payment decisions.

CHAPTER 8

Negotiating on Value

In Chapter 4, we described how the availability of information on healthcare value is supporting the increase in medical travel. This consumer-driven trend, while important, may not be as important as the effect that information about the value of healthcare may have on larger purchasers—employers, providers, payers, and policymakers. Here, too, trends overseas may indicate how the quest for higher-value care will unfold in the United States.

To define value, we first need to review some key economic concepts: costs, efficiency, effectiveness, comparative effectiveness, and cost-effectiveness. From a value perspective, *costs* include not only direct (accounting) costs but also opportunity costs. *Opportunity cost* is what you give up by making a decision, or your next best alternative. For example, if you decided to quit a full-time job to return to school, your direct costs would include tuition and books; your opportunity costs would include the salary and fringe benefits you would forgo while in school. When we measure value in healthcare, we need to include direct medical care and nonmedical care costs, as well as opportunity costs, in our cost calculations. *Efficiency* can refer to economic efficiency, which is attained when the treatment we choose is the least expensive among all possible treatments for the same condition. It can also refer to *technological efficiency*, which is achieved when the maximum possible improvement is attained from the set of inputs needed to produce the treatment. If we use more inputs than necessary to achieve a given level of health improvement, we are producing waste and are technologically inefficient. *Effectiveness* is the extent to which a treatment does what it was designed to do.

Comparative effectiveness and *cost-effectiveness* are relative terms used to compare one treatment to another. Comparative effectiveness is an evaluation of the effectiveness of a treatment relative to one or more alternative treatments. The National Institutes of Health defines comparative effectiveness as comparison of "the benefits and harms of different interventions and strategies to prevent, diagnose, treat and monitor health conditions in 'real world' settings" (Federal Coordinating Council for Comparative Effectiveness Research 2009). Cost-effectiveness is the link between efficiency and effectiveness and is determined by comparing the costs of alternative treatments to the effectiveness of alternative treatments.

There is a huge gap between the treatments used to address health conditions and the evidence we have of their value. The American Recovery and Reinvestment Act (ARRA) of 2009 and the Patient Protection and Affordable Care Act (PPACA) of 2010 allocated substantial resources to support comparative effectiveness research on surgeries, drugs, medical devices, and other treatments. The goal of these efforts is to identify and promote high-value treatment so that payers and policymakers can incentivize care that is (1) lower cost for the same quality level, (2) higher quality for the same cost, or (3) both higher quality and lower cost.

Although these approaches to evaluating care are substantially different from the approaches the United States has historically taken to evaluate care, they are not new. The United Kingdom in particular has been using some of these approaches for years. We can gain an understanding of how these approaches work and the effects they have on providers and payers by looking at their use in other countries.

THE ROLE OF HEALTH TECHNOLOGY ASSESSMENT IN OTHER COUNTRIES

The term *health technology assessment* refers to the processes used to evaluate a broad range of new healthcare technologies, including procedures, drugs, and medical devices. An assessment is a synthesis of existing scientific and nonscientific evidence, including information about safety, efficacy and effectiveness, and cost and cost-effectiveness (Sorenson, Drummond, and Kanavos 2008). Assessments focus on addressing four questions:

- *Effectiveness*: How well does the technology treat the condition?

- *Scope*: For what kinds of patients does the technology work?
- *Costs*: How much does it cost to use the technology?
- *Relation to existing technologies*: Does the technology perform better than, the same as, or worse than existing technologies?

In 2009, at least six countries had a formal health technology assessment process, but the roles of the evaluators and their evaluations differed. In some countries, the evaluator is an autonomous entity that simply does the evaluation and reports the results of the evaluation, while in other countries the evaluator is a member of the government, responsible for conducting evaluations and making decisions about coverage and pricing. Major countries with formal health technology assessment entities include the following (Sorenson, Drummond, and Kanavos 2008; Nasser and Sawicki 2009; Chalkidou 2009; Rochaix and Xerri 2009):

- Australia: Pharmaceutical Benefits Advisory Committee
- Finland: Finnish Office for Health Technology Assessment
- France: National Authority for Health

- Germany: Institute for Quality and Efficiency in Health Care
- Sweden: Swedish Council on Technology Assessment
- United Kingdom: National Institute for Health and Clinical Effectiveness (NICE)

Some countries, such as Australia, focus exclusively on drug effectiveness, while other countries' evaluations are more comprehensive and consider drugs, procedures, and medical devices (see Exhibit 8.1). In a number of cases, the entities conducting the assessments are of substantial size; however, their operating budgets are tiny in comparison to the savings realized from their decisions about the value of new technologies, which ultimately influence adoption and payment policies.

MORE SPENDING DOES NOT (NECESSARILY) MEAN BETTER OUTCOMES

There is both cross-country and within-country evidence that more spending does not necessarily translate into better outcomes, at least for many health conditions. Economists refer to this phenomenon as "flat-of-the-curve medicine."

EXHIBIT 8.1: Summary of National Entities

Country	Entity	Year of Inception	Annual Budget
Australia	Pharmaceutical Benefits Advisory Committee	Approx. 1989	$10M (2009–2010)
United Kingdom	National Institute for Health and Clinical Effectiveness	1999	$70M (2009)
France	National Authority for Health	2005	$97M (2008)
Germany	Institute for Quality and Efficiency in Health Care	2004	$21M (2009)

SOURCES: Chalkidou (2009); Lopert (2009); Nasser and Sawicki (2009); Rochaix and Xerri (2009).
NOTE: M = million.

That Conduct or Use Comparative Effectiveness Research for New Technologies

Structure	Purpose	Types of Evaluations	
		Procedures and Medical Devices	Drugs
Independent committee that makes advisory recommendations to government	To make coverage recommendations to government based on comparative effectiveness and comparative cost-effectiveness		Mandatory to add new drugs or new uses for existing drugs
A special health authority that makes recommendations to the National Health Service (NHS)	To reduce variation in practice, encourage dissemination of high-value innovations, and maximize health benefits for money spent by NHS	Mandatory	
Independent public organization that makes advisory recommendations to the Ministry of Health and Union of Sickness Funds	To conduct comparison of cost-effectiveness of individual technologies and groups of technologies or strategies	Mandatory for new technologies before they can be included on the public health insurance benefit list Multiple technology assessment (i.e., drug class or groups of medical devices or equipment) used for strategic and policy planning	
Independent body; advisory to Federal Joint Committee analysis only	To provide evidence-based evaluations of the costs and benefits of health services and make recommendations about coverage by the sickness funds	Covered for hospital procedures and medical devices, unless evaluation is negative; not covered for non-hospital procedures and devices, unless evaluation is positive	Covered unless explicit negative determination

For example, recent research has found that it is exceptionally difficult to increase life expectancy for certain conditions, even if money is no object (Rothberg et al. 2010); see Exhibit 8.2. For many conditions, inflation-adjusted cost increases have not yielded commensurate decreases in mortality. Between 2000 and 2004, hospital costs for acute myocardial infarction increased by 49 percent and for congestive heart failure by 60 percent, while mortality decreased by 21 percent and 19 percent respectively. Substantial differences were found in the cost per life year gained across different conditions and for different age groups. For example, the hospitalization costs per life year gained for acute myocardial infarction totaled $22,200 and for congestive heart failure totaled $201,600 for a person aged 55 to 65, but $98,200 and $100,900 respectively for a person aged 66 to 75. To successfully bend the cost curve and change the trajectory of healthcare spending, the United States needs to think critically about healthcare as a scarce resource (i.e., we do not have sufficient resources to provide an unlimited amount of healthcare) and how to optimally allocate this scarce resource.

In some countries, the body that assesses new technology will recommend against adopting a new technology if the incremental cost outweighs the incremental improvement it would make in health outcomes. For example, NICE recommended against National Health Service coverage of the bowel treatment drug Avastin (bevacizumab) for advanced bowel cancer treatment (McGrath 2010). NICE concluded that the cost of the drug was too high relative to the small increase in improvement it made over that realized through chemotherapy alone—a six-week increase in life expectancy at a cost of approximately $32,500 (Pidd 2010).

EDUCATING CONSUMERS ABOUT VALUE

The goal of health technology assessment is to make information accessible to purchasers and decision makers. As we inch toward a patient-centered care model in the United States, the patient will become an important consumer of this information. How will scientific evaluations be translated into materials that the lay consumer can use? As we discussed in Chapter 3, when talking about health and healthcare,

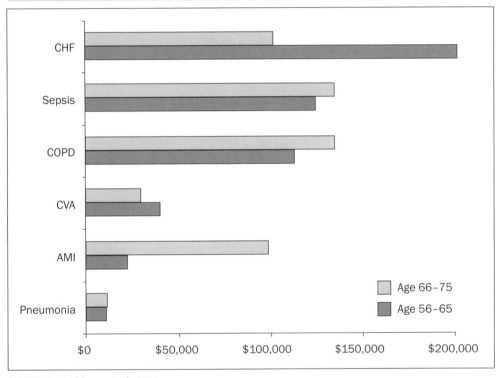

SOURCE: Rothberg et al. 2010.
NOTES: CHF = congestive heart failure; COPD = chronic obstructive pulmonary disease;
CVA = cerebral vascular accident (stroke); AMI = acute myocardial infarction.

providers and consumers use different terminology. Providers talk about their surgical procedures, while patients talk about their operations. When a primary care provider refers a patient to a cardiothoracic surgeon, the patient refers to the surgeon as a "heart doctor." Furthermore, evaluation of the scientific and nonscientific evidence about the effectiveness and value of a particular treatment is inherently complex; a treatment may work well for certain groups of patients but not for others. The evidence might be based only on clinical trials involving patients with no comorbid medical conditions, and therefore there may be no evidence about the effectiveness or cost-effectiveness of a treatment for patients with comorbid conditions, such as diabetes or heart disease.

Here, too, we can learn from models in other countries. The German Institute for Quality and Efficiency in Health Care, the entity charged with providing evidence-based evaluations of new health technologies, created a patient-focused website that translates its scientific evaluations into consumer-oriented materials (www.gesundheitsinformation .de/what-s-new.63.en.html) (Nasser and Sawicki 2009). NICE also uses a Web portal (www.evidence.nhs. uk) to disseminate evidence to key stakeholders, including patients and payers, but the portal is not tailored for use by the lay consumer (Chalkidou 2009).

A number of US providers and professional associations maintain websites full of medical information, such as Mayo Clinic (www .mayoclinic.org) and the American Academic of Family Physicians (www.familydoctor.org), but these sites do not synthesize the evidence regarding the effectiveness and value of alternative treatments for the lay consumer. For this information, consumers often turn to websites that contain health information provided by other consumers, such as Wikipedia (Abraham 2009). As consumer-driven healthcare grows and the demand for cost-effective treatments increases, a single reliable source that US consumers can turn to for assessments of procedures, medical devices, drugs, and other health information is likely to emerge. The most successful efforts will be those that communicate the evidence in language consumers can understand.

CONCLUSIONS

As the United States begins to systematically and objectively assess the effectiveness and value of alternative treatments, we will undoubtedly realize that we don't know as much as we thought we did about the effectiveness and value of care that is routinely provided. We will likely discover that the evidence is weak for some treatments that have been adopted as the "standard of care" and that the evidence for other treatments is surprisingly strong. The systematic assessment of treatments and the use of these results in value-based purchasing decisions will ultimately drive innovation in care delivery.

The United States can turn to other countries to learn what has and has not worked in systematic evaluations of new procedures, treatments, medical devices, and drugs at the national level. With access to an objective body of evidence, payers and providers can make more informed decisions. With access to evidence about value and effectiveness, consumers can examine their own values and weigh the trade-offs involved in these decisions.

The Numbers Behind the Trends

As the examples provided throughout this book illustrate, there are many sources of international comparisons and data on global trends. Many of these data sources are available online at no cost. In this appendix, we identify sources of data we have found particularly useful in studying and tracking global trends. Many industry associations also monitor trends and provide relevant data; our focus in this appendix is on sources that may be less familiar to readers.

Useful Sources of International Comparisons and Global Trends Data

Data	Source	Notes
Public health and health outcomes	Global InfoBase, World Health Organization https://apps.who.int/infobase	A rich source of cross-country health comparisons; includes tools for direct-country comparisons on public health, burden of disease, and mortality rates
Economics and health	Statistics Portal, Organisation for Economic Co-operation and Development (OECD) www.oecd.org/statistics	An extensive source of economic comparisons among developed countries, including comparisons of health and health systems; publishes free reports, white papers, and a subscription-based annual compendium of health data
Environmental/ climate change and health	World Resources Institute www.wri.org/publications/data-sets	Source of data and analyses concerning the effects of emerging and mature markets, environment, energy, and climate change, including health implications
Health system performance	The Commonwealth Fund www.commonwealthfund.org/ Content/Publications/Fund-Reports/ 2010/Jun/Mirror-Mirror-Update.aspx	A ranking-based index comparing US healthcare to six other developed countries on cost, quality, access, and efficiency; includes an interactive Web-based comparison tool
Information technology trends	Internet & American Life Project, Pew Research Center http://pewinternet.org	Reports, data sets, and other resources related to the Pew Research Center's ongoing research monitoring the impact of the Internet on work and home life; includes trends in Internet use for health-related purposes
Workforce trends	Global Atlas of the Health Workforce, World Health Organization http://apps.who.int/globalatlas/ default.asp	Provides geographic, age, and gender distributions of selected health professions within and across all countries that collect these data
	Health Workforce and Migration Project, OECD www.oecd.org/health/workforce	Provides longitudinal data on flows of foreign/foreign-trained doctors and nurses into OECD countries

Incorporating Global Trends Into Strategic Planning

Throughout this book we have described long-term trends through the lens of globalization and made the case that understanding these trends can help you help your organization capitalize on change rather than react to it. In this appendix, we describe a process by which these macro trends can be incorporated into the strategic planning process, using the experiences of CHRISTUS Health as our case study.

BACKGROUND

Although CHRISTUS Health traces its origins to the 1800s, its current structure was formed in 1999 through the acquisition of the assets of the Sisters of Charity of the Incarnate Word of Houston and the Incarnate Word Health System of San Antonio, making it one of the largest Catholic healthcare systems in the United States. Dr. Tom Royer became the new system's first CEO in 1999 and implemented its futures task force process shortly afterward. The primary goal of the futures task force is to ensure that macro and longer-term trends are appropriately influencing CHRISTUS's annual budget planning process and three-year budget forecasts. The output of the task force is a set of strategic directions that guides the three-year rolling strategic planning and budgeting process of the CHRISTUS system, regions, and business units. Not all implications influence the final plans, but by being aware of them, CHRISTUS Health and its components take a diligent look at the effect these forces may have on future strategy and operations.

When the formation of a futures task force was first proposed, it was difficult to sell the concept to the board and some senior leaders, given the challenges inherent in day-to-day operations and finance alone. Dr. Royer and his strategic planning team continue to champion its implementation, believing in the importance of devoting at least 5 percent of the energy of senior leadership and governance to considering what the next ten years will bring, regardless of how pressing the issues of the day may be. His 40 + years of experience in surgery has reinforced this belief, as he witnessed many disruptive changes related to medical advances that would have substantially cost the organizations he worked for had they not been evaluated strategically (e.g., needless expenditure on sunset technologies). His ability to provide these vivid examples helped him educate others on the importance of tracking such trends diligently.

THE FIRST FUTURES TASK FORCE: 2000–2001

The task force process proceeded through two phases. The first was a data-gathering phase. Participants developed a library of key resources—books and articles—for the team to read to get up to speed on the most interesting trends. The resources focused on trends that were larger than the organization ("looking from the outside in") and could affect operations down the road. Medical innovations; trends in areas such as population health, workforce, and government; and projections for the next 10 to 20 years were important parts of this research. Outside speakers regarded as visionaries who could be helpful to the group were also identified during this phase.

The second phase involved synthesizing this knowledge into implications. This work was accomplished over a series of five two-day meetings attended by the CEO, senior leaders, and the board, each held two to three months apart. The first part of this phase involved reviewing the readings and other materials and creating an array of "future facts"—elements of what the group thought the future would look like. Through this process, the group identified approximately 50 facts and then used them to identify what it saw as the key drivers of this envisioned future. The drivers identified at the time were disruptive and expensive technologies (e.g., robotic surgery, 64-slice CAT scans, the next generation of MRIs, artificial heart pumps), declining revenue (e.g., uninsurance/

underinsurance, increasing medical travel), and community-based care (e.g., outpatient procedures, technology-enabled independent living).

Four future scenarios were constructed on the basis of these drivers. From these scenarios, the group identified common themes and developed them into 19 recommendations. As a result of these recommendations, CHRISTUS decided to change its portfolio over time to one-third acute care, one-third non-acute care, and one-third international care. CHRISTUS also came to recognize that it needed to increase its federal advocacy as well as its emphasis on philanthropy.

THE SECOND FUTURES TASK FORCE: 2007–2008

By 2007, many findings from the original task force effort had become industry standard, diluting their strategic value to CHRISTUS. The environment had also changed substantially in response to global disruptive events and the changing political and economic landscape. Most important, the organization had arrived at another critical juncture in shaping its strategic direction and wanted to be sure that the long-term assumptions under which it was operating were correct. CHRISTUS began the second task force in October 2007.

In task force II, the group retained most of the structural elements from the original but also made several key changes. The first of these changes was to expand the group to include regional leaders. This extension was pursued because it made the process more inclusive and because the group thought the process had educational value for its participants. A second important change was to vary the locations of the meetings. All of the original task force's meetings were held in the Dallas area; the second task force's meetings were held as "learning journeys" in strategically selected locations around the world. To gain perspectives on medical travel and caring for the poor, the group held one of these meetings in India. To learn about models of socialized medicine, it held a meeting in Canada. To learn about recovery from a natural disaster, it held a meeting in New Orleans. The fourth meeting place, along the Texas/Mexico border, offered perspectives on transportation and care for the expanding base of the pyramid. The fifth meeting place, San Francisco (Silicon Valley), was chosen to gain insights into how emerging technologies were evolving to meet healthcare challenges. These efforts yielded 21 "future facts," which were used to identify new strategic directions (see Messbarger-Eguia 2009; Royer 2010).

CRITICAL ELEMENTS IN FUTURES PLANNING

The approach CHRISTUS Health has taken to futures planning works for its system, but it is only one approach, and variations may work better in some contexts. Regardless of the approach taken, the following three elements are critical to any futures planning process:

- *Environmental scan.* It is important to inform any futures planning process with a methodical consideration of multiple sources of trend information and to ensure that all participants have a chance to access and digest a common base of knowledge. Without this preparatory work, participants will be contributing mainly from their own fund of experience, which will tend to be focused from the "inside out"— how they see day-to-day operations evolving over time—rather than the "outside in"—how forces external to the organization will affect it in the future.

- *Reflective process*. A critical element of the meetings was the expectation that senior leaders spend time reflecting on the present and future context in which their organizations operate. Senior leaders should devote at least 5 percent of their energy on an ongoing basis to learning about these longer-term environmental trends. By creating a futures task force and setting a meeting schedule, they explicitly incorporate this work into their calendars. This process also needs to be structured effectively to ensure that the group reaches consensus on a specific set of implications that will inform the strategic planning process.

- *Systematic use of results*. Futures planning is only as useful as it is actionable. The use of futures planning results needs to be structured into the organization's regular strategic and budgetary planning processes. If the results do not become an explicit part of the strategic plan, they still should be used to test assumptions in budget planning and forecasting.

References

Abraham, L. 2010. "Key Trends in the Digital World: Focus on Government, Health, Travel, and e-Commerce." Presentation at Measuring and Enhancing Services Trade Data and Information Conference, US Department of Commerce, Washington, DC, September 14.

———. 2009. "Innovation in the Collection and Dissemination of Data." Presentation at Measuring and Enhancing Services Trade Data and Information Conference, US Department of Commerce, Washington, DC, September 14.

American Hospital Association. 2009. "Fast Facts on US Hospitals." www.aha.org/aha/resource-center/Statistics-and-Studies/fast-facts.html.

American Medical Association. 2010. "International Graduates in American Medicine: Contemporary Challenges and Opportunities." www.ama-assn.org/ama1/pub/upload/mm/18/img-workforce-paper.pdf.

Appleby, J. 2010. "Domestic Medical Travel Is Taking Off for Surgery Deals." *USA Today,* July 9. www.usatoday.com/money/industries/health/2010-07-07-travelforhealth07_CV_N.htm.

Arai, H. 2009. "Geriatrics in the Most Aged Country, Japan." *Archives of Gerontology and Geriatrics* 49 (suppl. 2): S1–2.

Bauer, J. C. 2009. "Medical Tourism: Wave of the Future in a World of Hurt?" *Healthcare Financial Management* 63 (8): 36–38, 40, 42.

Bodenheimer, T., E. Chen, and H. D. Bennett. 2009. "Confronting the Growing Burden of Chronic Disease: Can the US Health Care Workforce Do the Job?" *Health Affairs (Millwood)* 28 (1): 64–74.

Byron, E. 2007. "P&G's Global Target: Shelves of Tiny Stores." *Wall Street Journal*, July 16. http://online.wsj.com/article/SB118454911342967244.html.

Campbell, J. C., N. Ikegami, and M. J. Gibson. 2010. "Lessons from Public Long-Term Care Insurance in Germany and Japan." *Health Affairs (Millwood)* 29 (1): 87–95.

Carman, K. L., M. Maurer, J. M. Yegian, P. Dardess, J. McGee, M. Evers, and K. O. Marlo. 2010. "Evidence That Consumers Are Skeptical About Evidence-Based Health Care." *Health Affairs (Millwood)* 29 (7): 1400–406.

Central Intelligence Agency. 2010. *The World Factbook*. https://www.cia.gov/library/publications/the-world-factbook/index.html.

Chalkidou, K. 2009. "Comparative Effectiveness Review Within the UK's National Institute for Health and Clinical Excellence." Commonwealth Fund publication 1296, volume 59. www.commonwealthfund.org/~/media/Files/Publications/Issue%20Brief/2009/Jul/Chalkidou/1296_Chalkidou_UK_CER_issue_brief_717.pdf.

Christensen, C. M., R. Bohmer, and J. Kenagy. 2000. "Will Disruptive Innovations Cure Health Care?" *Harvard Business Review* 78 (5): 102–12.

Claxton, G., B. DiJulio, B. Finder, J. Lundy, M. McHugh, A. Osei-Anto, H. Whitmore, J. Pickreign, and J. Gabel. 2010. "Employer Health Benefits 2010 Annual Survey." Menlo Park, CA, and Chicago: The Henry J. Kaiser Family Foundation and Health Research & Educational Trust. http://ehbs.kff.org/pdf/2010/8085.pdf.

Cleveland Clinic. 2010. "Lowe's Expands Heart Healthcare Benefits with Cleveland Clinic." February 16. http://my.clevelandclinic.org/news/2010/lowes_expands_heart_healthcare_benefits.aspx.

Cooperman, S. 2007. "Patient Travelers." *Forbes,* October 29. www.forbes.com/forbes-life -magazine/2007/1029/095.html.

Cortez, N. 2009. "International Health Care Convergence: The Benefits and Burdens of Market-Driven Standardization." *Wisconsin International Law Journal* 26 (3): 646–704.

D'Aunno, T., J. R. Kimberly, and G. de Pouvourville. 2008. "Conclusions: The Global Diffusion of Casemix." In *The Globalization of Managerial Innovation in Health Care,* edited by J. R. Kimberly, G. de Pouvourville, and T. D'Aunno, 346–72. New York: Cambridge University Press.

DeNavas-Walt, C., B. D. Proctor, and J. C. Smith, US Census Bureau. 2010. Current Population Reports, P60-238: "Income, Poverty, and Health Insurance Coverage in the United States: 2009." Washington, DC: US Government Printing Office. www.census.gov/prod/2010pubs/ p60-238.pdf.

Dill, M. J., and E. S. Salsberg. 2008. "The Complexities of Physician Supply and Demand: Projections Through 2025." Center for Workforce Studies. https://services.aamc.org/ publications/showfile.cfm?file = version122.pdf&prd_id = 244&prv_id = 299&pdf_id = 122.

Ehrbeck, T., C. Guevara, and P. D. Mango. 2008. "Mapping the Market for Medical Tourism." *McKinsey Quarterly,* May. www.mckinseyquarterly.com/Mapping_the_market_for_travel_2134.

Federal Coordinating Council for Comparative Effectiveness Research. 2009. "Report to the President and the Congress, June 30, 2009." Washington, DC: US Department of Health and Human Services. www.hhs.gov/recovery/programs/cer/cerannualrpt.pdf.

Fox, S., and S. Jones. 2009. "The Social Life of Health Information." Washington, DC: Pew Internet & American Life Project. www.pewinternet.org/ ~ /media//Files/Reports/2009/PIP_ Health_2009.pdf.

Freyer, F. J. 2007. "Outsourcing to India Hip Surgery." *The Providence Journal,* June 22. www.projo.com/travel/content/MEDICAL_TOURISM_06-24-07_AE617S5.1f0d20d.html.

Fujisawa, R., and G. Lafortune. 2007. "The Remuneration of General Practitioners and Specialists in 14 OECD Countries: What Are the Factors Influencing Variations Across Countries?" OECD Health Working Papers No.41. www.oecd.org/dataoecd/51/48/41925333.pdf.

Garman, A. N., A. Milstein, and M. Anderson. 2008. "Medical Travel." In *Encyclopedia of Health Services Research*, edited by R. M. Mullner, 744–46. Thousand Oaks, CA: Sage.

Hammond, A., W. J. Kramer, J. Tran, R. Katz, and C. Walker. 2007. *The Next 4 Billion: Market Size and Business Strategy at the Base of the Pyramid*. Washington, DC: World Resource Institute.

Hartwig, I., and P. Nicolaides. 2003. "Elusive Solidarity in an Enlarged European Union." *Eipascope* 3: 19–25.

ICH. 2000. "History and Future of ICH." www.ich.org/cache/compo/276-254-1.html.

IIE Network. 2010. *Open Doors Report 2010*. www.iie.org/en/Research-and-Publications/Open-Doors.

Immelt, J. R., V. Govindarajan, and C. Trimble. 2009. "How GE Is Disrupting Itself." *Harvard Business Review* (October): 56–65.

International Monetary Fund. 2010. "World Economic Outlook October 2010: Recovery, Risk, and Rebalancing." www.imf.org/external/pubs/ft/weo/2010/02/pdf/text.pdf.

Johnson, T. J., and A. N. Garman. 2010. "Impact of Medical Travel on Imports and Exports of Medical Services." *Health Policy* 98 (2–3): 171–77.

Joint Commission International. 2010. "Joint Commission International (JCI) Accredited Organizations." www.jointcommissioninternational.org/JCI-Accredited-Organizations.

Kaiser Family Foundation. 2010. "Survey of People Who Purchase Their Own Insurance." June. Menlo Park, CA: The Henry J. Kaiser Family Foundation. www.kff.org/kaiserpolls/upload/8077-R.pdf.

———. 2008. "Economic Problems Facing Families." Survey brief, April. Menlo Park, CA: The Henry J. Kaiser Family Foundation. www.kff.org/kaiserpolls/upload/7773.pdf.

Keckley, P. H., and H. R. Underwood. 2008. "Medical Tourism: Consumers in Search of Value." Deloitte Center for Health Solutions. www.deloitte.com/assets/Dcom-Croatia/Local%20Assets/Documents/hr_Medical_tourism(3).pdf.

Lopert, R. 2009. "Evidence-Based Decision-Making Within Australia's Pharmaceutical Benefits Scheme." Commonwealth Fund publication 1297, volume 60. www.commonwealthfund.org/~/media/Files/Publications/Issue%20Brief/2009/Jul/Chalkidou/1297_Lopert_CER_Australia_issue_brief_724.pdf.

McGrath, S. 2010. "UK Regulator Rejects Roche's Avastin Again." *Wall Street Journal,* August 24. http://online.wsj.com/article/SB10001424052748703447004575448902831710956.html.

Medical Tourism Association. 2010. "Medical Tourism Sample Surgery Cost Chart." Updated in June. West Palm Beach, FL. www.medicaltourismassociation.com/userfiles/files/Pricing%20 Chart%202010.pdf.

Messbarger-Eguia, A. P. 2009. "Facing the Future: The CHRISTUS Health Futures Task Force II." Presentation to the Texas Healthcare Financial Management Association, March. www.hfmatexas.org/files/file/Documents/Presentations/Messbarger_Facing_the_Future_The_ CHRISTUS_Health_futures_3up.ppt.pdf.

Milstein, A., and M. Smith. 2007. "Will the Surgical World Become Flat?" *Health Affairs* 26 (1): 137–41.

Nasser, M., and P. Sawicki. 2009. "Institute for Quality and Efficiency in Health Care: Germany." Commonwealth Fund publication 1294, volume 57. www.commonwealthfund .org/~/media/Files/Publications/Issue%20Brief/2009/Jul/Chalkidou/1294_Nasser_CER_ Germany_issue_brief_724.pdf.

Newsome, B. 2008. "Patients with Passports: More Opting to Go Abroad for Surgery." *Colorado Springs Gazette,* July 14.

Nexon, D., and S. J. Ubl. 2010. "Implications of Health Reform for the Medical Technology Industry." *Health Affairs (Millwood)* 29 (7): 1325–29.

Organisation for Economic Co-operation and Development (OECD). 2010a. "Growing Health Spending Puts Pressure on Government Budgets, According to OECD Health Data 2010." www.oecd.org/document/11/0,3343,en_21571361_44315115_45549771_1_1_1_1,00.html.

————. 2010b. "Country Statistical Profiles 2010: Germany." http://stats.oecd.org/index .aspx?queryid = 23071.

————. 2010c. *OECD Health Data 2010.* Paris, France: Organisation for Economic Co-operation and Development.

————. 2010d. "OECD Health Data 2010—Country Notes and Press Releases." www.oecd.org/do cument/46/0,3343,en_2649_34631_34971438_1_1_1_1,00.html.

————. 2008. "The Looming Crisis in the Health Workforce: How Can OECD Countries Respond?" www.who.int/hrh/migration/looming_crisis_health_workforce.pdf.

Peterson, C. L., and R. Burton. 2007. "CRS Report for Congress: US Health Care Spending: Comparison with Other OECD Countries." Washington, DC: Congressional Research Service. http://assets.opencrs.com/rpts/RL34175_20070917.pdf.

Pidd, H. 2010. "Avastin Prolongs Life but Drug Is Too Expensive for NHS Patients, Says NICE." *The Guardian,* August 24. www.guardian.co.uk/society/2010/aug/24/avastin-too-expensive -for-patients.

Rechel, B., Y. Doyle, E. Grundy, and M. McKee. 2009. "Policy Brief 10: How Can Health Systems Respond to Population Ageing?" Copenhagen, Denmark: World Health Organization. www.euro.who.int/__data/assets/pdf_file/0004/64966/E92560.pdf.

Rochaix, L., and B. Xerri. 2009. "National Authority for Health: France." Commonwealth Fund publication 1295, volume 58. www.commonwealthfund.org/ ~ /media/Files/Publications/ Issue%20Brief/2009/Jul/Chalkidou/1295_Rochaix_CER_France_issue_brief_724.pdf.

Rogers, E. M. 1995. *Diffusion of Innovations,* fourth edition. New York: Free Press.

Rothberg, M. B., J. Cohen, P. Lindenauer, J. Maselli, and A. Auerbach. 2010. "Little Evidence of Correlation Between Growth in Health Care Spending and Reduced Mortality." *Health Affairs (Millwood)* 29 (8): 1523–31.

Rothberg, M. B., E. Morsi, E. M. Benjamin, P. S. Pekow, and P. K. Lindenauer. 2008. "Choosing the Best Hospital: The Limitations of Public Quality Reporting." *Health Affairs (Millwood)* 27 (6): 1680–87.

Royer, T. 2010. "Findings of CHRISTUS' Second Futures Task Force." Weblog post, May 5. http://wiresidechatwithdrtom.blogspot.com/2010/03/findings-of-christus-second-futures.html.

Satjapot, S. P., T. J. Johnson, and A. N. Garman. 2011. "International Medical Travelers, Length of Stay, and the Continuum of Care: Inquiry and Comparison." *Quality Management in Health Care* 20 (1): 76–83.

Shortell, S. M., L. P. Casalino, and E. S. Fisher. 2010. "How the Center for Medicare and Medicaid Innovation Should Test Accountable Care Organizations." *Health Affairs (Millwood)* 29 (7): 1293–98.

Smith, S., J. P. Newhouse, and M. S. Freeland. 2009. "Income, Insurance, and Technology: Why Does Health Spending Outpace Economic Growth?" *Health Affairs (Millwood)* 28 (5): 1276–84.

Sorenson, C., M. Drummond, and P. Kanavos. 2008. "Ensuring Value for Money in Health Care: The Role of Health Technology Assessment in the European Union." European Observatory on Health Systems and Policies, Observatory Studies Series No. 11. Copenhagen, Denmark: World Health Organization. www.euro.who.int/__data/assets/pdf_file/0011/98291/E91271.pdf.

University HealthSystem Consortium. 2010. "About UHC." https://www.uhc.edu/12443.htm.

US Census Bureau. 2008. Table 2: "Projections of the Population by Selected Age Groups and Sex for the United States: 2010 to 2050"; and Table 4: "Projections of the Population by Sex, Race, and Hispanic Origin for the United States: 2010 to 2050." www.census.gov/population/ www/projections/summarytables.html.

US Department of Commerce, International Trade Administration Office of Travel & Tourism Industries. 2010. "Survey of International Air Travelers Program." http://tinet.ita.doc.gov/research/programs/ifs/examples.html.

US Department of Health and Human Services, Office of Inspector General. 2010. "Challenges to FDA's Ability to Monitor and Inspect Foreign Clinical Trials." http://oig.hhs.gov/oei/reports/oei-01-08-00510.pdf.

Wooldridge, A. 2010. "The Power to Disrupt: Business Innovations from Emerging Markets Will Change the Rich World Too." *The Economist* (April 17): 12–14.

Woodman, J. 2007. *Patients Beyond Borders: Everybody's Guide to Affordable, World-Class Medical Tourism*. Chapel Hill, NC: Healthy Travel Media.

About the Authors

Andrew N. Garman, PsyD, is associate chair of the Department of Health Systems Management at Rush University Medical Center and chief executive officer of the National Center for Healthcare Leadership in Chicago. Over the past several years, he has collaborated with Tricia Johnson on several projects investigating patterns in international travel for medical care, including an industry studies project funded by the Alfred P. Sloan Foundation. With support from the US Department of Commerce and in collaboration with the University HealthSystem Consortium, this work has expanded into assessment and analysis of trends in the health services trade.

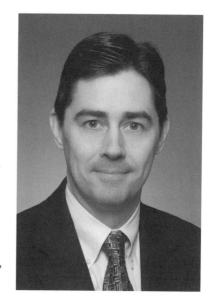

Dr. Garman is a recognized authority in evidence-based leadership assessment and development. He is coauthor of two books, *Exceptional Leadership* and *The Healthcare C-Suite: Leadership Development at the Top* (Health Administration Press), as well as several dozen peer-reviewed research articles and book chapters. For his studies of leadership competencies and CEO succession planning, he is a three-time recipient of the American College of Healthcare Executives Health Management Research Award. A frequently requested keynote speaker and workshop leader, he also consults with executives and their organizations on their leadership development and people management strategies.

Dr. Garman's professional experience includes a variety of practitioner and faculty roles in major institutions, including the Federal Reserve Bank of Chicago, Illinois Institute of Technology, University of Chicago, and Illinois Department of Mental Health. He received his BS in psychology/mathematics from Penn State, his MS in personnel and human resource development from Illinois Institute of Technology, and his PsyD in clinical psychology from the College of William & Mary/Virginia Consortium. He is also an Illinois-licensed clinical psychologist and a senior fellow with the Health Research and Educational Trust.

Tricia J. Johnson, PhD, is associate professor in the Department of Health Systems Management and director of the Center for Health Management and Policy Research at Rush University in Chicago. Dr. Johnson is a leader in forecasting trends in healthcare innovation and globalization and predicting the ways in which innovations in quality, safety, and efficiency will shape the future of healthcare. In collaboration with the University Health-System Consortium, she and Dr. Garman are leading the evaluation of a US Department of Commerce–funded initiative to increase the number of international patients traveling to the United States for medical care. Drs. Johnson and Garman recently completed a project 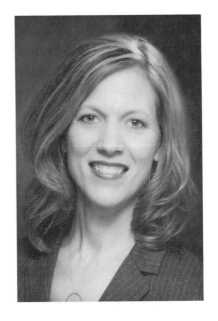 that examined trends in international medical travel and the implications of those trends for US providers. They are also the authors of a blog on medical travel research (http://medicaltravelresearch.wordpress.com).

As a health economist, her research focuses on economic and policy issues related to consumers and healthcare providers, including innovation, globalization, the effect of economic incentives on behavior, and the cost and cost-effectiveness of hospital and community-based interventions to improve the quality of health and healthcare. Her work has been funded by the National Institutes of Health, Cardinal Health Foundation, Alfred P. Sloan Foundation, World Bank and Albanian Ministry of Health, and US Department of Commerce. Dr. Johnson was a 2008–2009 Fulbright Scholar in Austria, where she worked with faculty in the Institute for Social Policy at the Vienna University of Economics and Business.

Dr. Johnson earned her BA in economics and business administration from Coe College in Cedar Rapids, Iowa, her MA in hospital and health administration from The University of Iowa, and her MS and PhD in economics from Arizona State University in Tempe.

Thomas C. Royer, MD, is chief executive officer and president of the CHRISTUS Health system, where he leads day-to-day operations and lends extensive expertise in developing physician partnerships and community health programs. In his nearly seven years with the organization, Dr. Royer has led CHRISTUS Health through a remarkable period of growth, making it one of the ten largest Catholic health systems in the United States today. In 2006 and 2007, he was named the seventh most powerful physician executive in healthcare by *Modern Physician* magazine.

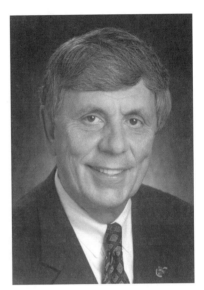

Prior to joining CHRISTUS, Dr. Royer served as chairman of the board of governors for the Henry Ford Medical Group and senior vice president of medical affairs for the Henry Ford Health System. In addition to leading major operations, Dr. Royer was instrumental in developing physician partnerships and community health programs and services and introducing alternative and complementary medicine at Henry Ford.

In addition to his experience with Henry Ford, Dr. Royer served for two years at Johns Hopkins Medical Services Corporation and Wyman Park Medical Associates in Baltimore in a variety of positions, including chief executive officer, president and chief operating officer, and vice president of clinical operations. He also spent 18 years with Geisinger Medical Center and Clinic in Danville, Pennsylvania, as senior vice president and medical director after founding the Center's department of emergency medicine, emergency medicine residency program, and Susquehanna Poison Control Program.

In August 2005, Dr. Royer was invited to represent CHRISTUS Health as one of 350 delegates at the fifth Forbes Global CEO Conference held in Sydney, Australia. As the only physician and CEO of a nonprofit, multi-geographic healthcare system, Dr. Royer was asked to participate in a workshop to discuss the complex issues the healthcare industry is facing and the leadership characteristics required to facilitate significant change in measurable benchmark goals.

Dr. Royer has been published in numerous medical and trade publications, including the *Health Forum Journal, Medical Group Management Association Journal, Physician Executive Journal, Deloitte Review,* and *Crossroads* (Deloitte). Dr. Royer, who is board-certified in surgery, received his medical degree from the University of Pennsylvania and completed his postdoctoral training at Geisinger Medical Center and Clinic.

Additional resources from Andrew Garman and Health Administration Press

Exceptional Leadership: 16 Critical Competencies for Healthcare Executives
Carson F. Dye, FACHE, and Andrew N. Garman, PsyD

There are good leaders, then there are exceptional leaders. The answer to "What makes a leader exceptional?" is simple: competencies. Competencies are a set of professional and personal skills, knowledge, values, and traits that guide a leader's performance.

This book focuses on the 16 key competencies that distinguish good leadership from great leadership.

The Healthcare C-Suite: Leadership Development at the Top
Andrew N. Garman, PsyD, and Carson F. Dye, FACHE

Leadership development at the executive level requires a different approach. Learn what senior executives can do to help others harness, strengthen, and optimize their talents and capabilities.

This book offers strategies for overcoming common barriers to leadership development at the C-suite level that can lead to ongoing blind spots and unrealized potential.

For more information or to purchase these books, visit our online bookstore at ache.org.hap

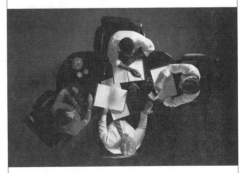